ITCH.
SCRATCH.
REPEAT.

A Memoir of Overcoming Eczema

CLAIRE R. KENEALLY, MA, AHIP

EXASPERATING

CHRONIC

ZAPPING

EMBARRASSING

MISUNDERSTOOD

AGONIZING

CONTENTS

PART TWO

FOREWORD

ECZEMA IS EVERYWHERE. Television commercials appear daily, promoting new treatments. Magazine and newspaper ads from pharmaceutical companies beg eczema sufferers to enroll in drug trials. Pharmacy aisles are jam-packed with creams, ointments, sprays, and other items offering help to treat eczema.

Eczema, sometimes called atopic dermatitis, is on the rise. According to an article in *Annals of Nutrition and Metabolism*, eczema/atopic dermatitis "affects 15-20% of children and 1 to 3% of adults worldwide." This means that a lot of people are tormented by this confounding, irritating, and incurable condition. While certainly not life threatening, it does affect one's quality of life.

Friends complain about having the condition and not being able to get rid of it. I can relate. I had eczema for most of my life, decades in fact. Many times, eczema occurs in infancy and then disappears, but mine arrived at the age of eight as I sat quietly in my third-grade classroom. My left hand started to itch uncontrollably, and thus began the lifelong ritual of "Itch. Scratch. Repeat."

Eczema treatment has changed very little since I was diagnosed with it in the 1960s. A tube of steroid cream was the standard fix for this frustrating condition. This remedy did not work for me. An article in *JAMA Dermatology* makes the bold statement that "Atopic dermatitis is probably a life-long illness."

Eczema slowly and silently sneaked into many areas of my life, something I certainly didn't expect as I scratched my hand that first time so long ago. It subtly influenced my career choices, where I would live, and the hobbies I would enjoy. It boldly affected the foods I would eat, the soaps I would use, and the clothing I would wear. Most of the time it resided somewhat peacefully in the background of my life, annoying but tolerable. Occasionally it would take center stage, rising to a fury as I tried to control it. During those trying times, the sleepless nights, unbearable itching, and bloody hands became the focus of my life. The quest for relief was all I could think about. It effectively and completely took over my life. Eczema was winning the battles, but as the saying goes, not the war.

I eventually conquered it and wanted to share my story in the event it might help others. I must clarify that this book is a memoir about living with a common skin condition. It is not a medical advice book, nor does it contain long lists of treatments or regimens that one should try. I am a medical librarian, not a physician. However, I have provided a selective medical literature search in Part Two of this book to enlighten the reader on the difficulties inherent in treating eczema.

I also took the liberty of sharing anecdotes from my life that are in some way related to eczema, and in truth to make the book a bit more interesting and readable. I hope that those with eczema will relate to my musings and know they are not alone. I should also state that my severe case of eczema was primarily on my hands. It did occasionally gravitate to other body parts, but it was always predominately hand eczema. Intense, uncontrollable itching was the main symptom of my case.

It is my wish that what ultimately "cured" my eczema might work for others, though the medical literature is certainly divided on the issue.

So, for now, sit back, relax, and stop scratching long enough to read a few pages.

PART ONE

PROLOGUE

I AM STANDING in a brightly lit cosmetics store at a large, bustling mall in Tampa, Florida. On this beautiful winter day in February 2010, I am excited to be here as I admire the vast array of scented body lotions, shower gels, and soaps. I am deciding which ones to buy and am overwhelmed with choices, but mostly I am just happy to be here. To the average person, this would be no big deal, certainly not worth writing about, but for me this is huge. This is one of the first days of my new life – a life without chronic hand eczema. After suffering for over forty-five years, I am finally free of it. And, after being told by countless doctors that I should only use certain special products on my skin and avoid anything scented, perfumed, or for that matter just about anything other than a mild soap, I can use whatever I wish. At the age of fifty-four, I now have normal skin just like everyone else.

The days of endless scratching, sleepless nights, and blood on the sheets are over. I think back to the time when it all started. I was a shy, obedient child growing up in Gloversville, a tiny town in upstate New York, when one cold winter day my left hand started to itch…

JUMPING OFF

Chapter 1

THREE THINGS HAPPENED the year I turned eight. We moved to a new neighborhood, I developed eczema on my hands, and my father got lung cancer.

It was the summer of 1963 when we rented the new apartment, just two blocks from our old one in Gloversville, New York, a small town in the foothills of the Adirondack mountains. Our new apartment was on the second floor of the house, upstairs from the landlords, just like the other one, but it was bigger and had two living rooms in the front. One of them had to be used as a bedroom because my parents' bedroom furniture would not fit into either of the small bedrooms. I got my own tiny bedroom off the dining room. It had a large, gold-colored radiator where my mother would warm my school clothes on cold upstate New York mornings. The place was drafty, and the radiators creaked as they struggled to heat the rooms.

I loved it there at first. I had a whole new group of kids to play with. My best friend was Danny. He was three years younger than I, which made him only five when our friendship began. But he was nicer than his brothers and sisters. I should have been hanging around with his older sister who was closer to my age, but she was part of the neighborhood clique, a group into which I would never quite fit.

That first summer Danny and I played kickball, rode our bikes, and caroused the neighborhood. When it rained, we played board games in the kitchen nook at the back of his house.

Danny's house was big, and much nicer than our upstairs flat. On top of that, his family owned it. The house had lots of bedrooms and a big playroom stuffed with the latest toys. That summer they bought the very best thing ever, a trampoline for their backyard. Their house became a magnet for all the neighborhood children. So many kids wanted to jump on it that they finally brought out a timer, so it would be fair and everyone would get the same amount of time to jump.

Danny's older brother and sister taught me how to do a front flip. They were excited for me when I mastered it. I loved the trampoline. We jumped every day, all day. Danny's parents were happy that the trampoline was such a hit, but as time went on, they became concerned that someone might get hurt. We always had spotters when we jumped, one person on each side of the trampoline, but especially at each end. We weren't supposed to jump without this safety precaution.

One month after the trampoline arrived, Danny's dad made each child's parents sign a waiver that they would not sue if a fall or injury should occur. I was afraid that my parents wouldn't sign it. They were a bit overprotective, my mother mostly. They knew how much I loved it, so my dad finally signed it after some serious begging on my part. I never fell off or got hurt, but I did hit the springs a couple of times. Of course, I never told them about the near misses.

The trampoline was the very best thing about that summer. It was the calm before the storm.

ITCH. SCRATCH. REPEAT.

Chapter 2

THE TEMPERATURE WAS in the low thirties the morning it started. On that typical, upstate New York winter day in March 1964, I walked the half mile to school as I usually did. I loved school and especially my third-grade teacher, Mrs. Williams. She was an older lady with gray hair in a bun and heavy beaded jewelry. Her colorful necklace clanked on my desk every time she checked my work. She was very kind to me because I was a good student and always obedient.

We were doing some arithmetic when it first began. My left hand started to itch. I scratched it. It itched more. I scratched more. I stopped doing my work. Mrs. Williams didn't notice, thank goodness. I always wanted to please her. I looked at my hands and there were little bubbles on my palm. The bubbles popped when I scratched them. A clear liquid came out. The itching stopped after a couple of minutes and my hands looked normal again. I forgot about it and finished my arithmetic problems. Mrs. Williams never knew anything had happened.

On the walk home from school my hand started to itch again. The day had grown colder and the wind was blowing hard. My left hand was really itching, even worse than before. I scratched under my wooly mitten, but that wasn't enough. I finally took the mitten off and rubbed my hand against my jacket. It was very cold now and my hand was freezing but the itching was worse. I had to make it stop. I rubbed and scratched and rubbed again. The bubbles were back and they seemed bigger. The palm of my hand was red. I was uncomfortable, but the worst was yet to come.

Walking up behind me was Danny's sister Susan and her best friend, Mary. Susan saw that my mitten was off, so she snatched it out of my hand and threw it in the snowbank. Mary grabbed my other mitten, pulled it off, and threw it in the road. I ran to grab the first one, but Susan beat me to it and tossed that one in the road. I stumbled over the snowbank to retrieve them, but it was two against one. They were each holding one of my mittens and taunting me, "Come and get them, Claire, come and get them."

This was a game I could not win. I walked on without my mittens. When I neared my house, they walked past me and threw the mittens down on the sidewalk. I was afraid to pick them up, figuring it would all start again. But they must have been bored with the game, as they continued on without even looking at me. I hated the negative attention, but I hated being ignored even more. When they were a good distance ahead, I picked up my mittens from the icy ground and sprinted for home. On the bright side, I had forgotten all about my itchy hand.

FIRST DOC

Chapter 3

I WAS SITTING cross-legged on the floor in the front living room when my mother first saw me scratching. She bent over me to see what I was doing, and I caught a look of concern on her face. It would be the first of many times she would look at my hands and worry. My hands did not hurt; they simply itched, so I was okay with it. Clearly my mother was not, and she made an appointment with my pediatrician right away. I had been going to him since I was three or four. I did not particularly like him, because I usually got a shot when I went to his office. I hoped this time would be different.

My pediatrician referred me to a local dermatologist, who we saw later in the week. That dermatology appointment would be the first of many, and quietly set the stage for a firestorm of disappointments. I had to miss school to go to the appointment, which I hated. I did not want to fall behind in my work, but even more importantly, I did not want the other kids asking why I was not at school. I got along with my classmates better than with the neighborhood kids, but I still didn't want to share details of the rather unpleasant turn of events.

The dermatologist took a quick look at my hands and stated that I had eczema, a common skin condition. He prescribed a steroid cream and told me to rub it on my hands, but only on the parts that itched. I was terrified that the cream would hurt, and I did not want to follow his orders. After we got home, my mother helped me rub it on my hands, just on the red spots where I had been scratching. It burned a bit and I started to cry.

"This cream will make it all better," she consoled me. "It will make it go completely away," she repeated.

I am certain that my mother did not realize she had just told me a big fat lie. This was the first of many falsehoods about eczema that I would hear throughout my life. Nonetheless, I believed my mother and truly expected the steroid cream to fix the problem permanently. I added the word "eczema" to my third-grade vocabulary and set off on a journey that would last decades, though I certainly didn't know it at the time.

After a few days of using the steroid cream, the eczema did go away. I was happy it was gone and promptly forgot about it. But, two weeks later, it was back. This was puzzling to my mother and especially to me. I had not been sick much in my young life. A short bout of the flu at the age of six and an occasional cold were my only complaints. I had not even had the typical childhood illnesses like chicken pox, measles, or mumps. I had never broken a bone or even had a cavity filled in my teeth.

If I did get a cold, it would go away after a few days. It did not come back. When I fell and scraped my knee, it healed. The scrape did not suddenly reappear. I was confused and wondered why the itching and rash were coming back. My mother was puzzled also. Nonetheless, she continued to rub the cream on my hands faithfully for the next month, but the itching persisted. When we went back to the dermatologist I was given a stronger steroid cream, which, like the first one, didn't do much. I continued to question why the eczema wasn't going away, and as I wondered, I kept on scratching my hands whenever they itched.

When my classmates saw me scratching, I told them it was eczema. This was a good enough explanation for most of them.

Danny, however, seemed concerned at first. "Can I catch it?" he asked. "No!" I replied firmly, not wanting to lose a good friend over a stupid rash. After thinking for a moment, he nodded his head in agreement.

DEFEETED

Chapter 4

WHEN THE SCHOOL year ended in June, I looked forward to summer vacation. Even in typically cold upstate New York, there were some beautiful sunny warm days at that time of year and the neighborhood kids were playing outside a lot, myself included. Things were heating up in the neighborhood in more ways than one. Barb, who lived two blocks over, had become good friends with Susan and Mary, the ones who had stolen my mittens. Barb had an older brother, Lee, who was starting to come around too. Lively kickball games began in the backyard of Danny's house. The group of neighborhood kids got larger and larger. It was great fun, and as an only child I reveled in this big group of potential playmates. But they were mostly older and louder. I was just a quiet, tiny girl who happened to live there. I had no brothers or sisters who had my back. My two cousins were older so we never played together. I had to make the best of the situation.

There were good days and bad days. On a good day, they encouraged me when I kicked the ball well and cheered as I ran around the bases. It felt good, like the earlier times when they taught me the front flip on the trampoline. I was so happy to fit in with them. But my joy did not last long. The very next day they would tell me I could not play because I was too young or too small or just not good enough.

Some days they ignored me as if I were invisible. The rejection hurt and I did not understand it. I hadn't done anything to them. When I complained to my mother, she told me to just ignore it. And sure enough, the next day they would be nice again. It was so weird and unpredictable, just like my eczema.

They started making fun of the way my mother would call for me when it was time for dinner. In those days it was safe for children to roam the neighborhood and I thoroughly enjoyed this wonderful freedom. I was a conscientious child and my mother knew I would not go too far. When it was dinnertime, mom would stand on the back porch and call out my name until I would answer, "Coming!" This worked great for us, until the teasing began.

"Claire, Claire, Claire," they taunted in a sing-song voice, contorting their faces with every word. Each evening when my mother called out my name, I counted the seconds until their mocking began. "Claire, Claire, Claire," the ritual continued. I hated it and I was starting to hate them. I still hung with Danny. He was never mean, ever. We rode our bikes and played our board games, but how I wanted to fit in with the big group! It just wasn't meant to be.

I was almost nine and had been fighting the eczema for nearly six months. Like the kids in the neighborhood, it was erratic – good on some days and downright nasty on other days. I had gotten used to the steroid cream and could rub it on my hands myself without my mother's help. But when my hands itched, I scratched them. That is all there was to it. I continued to scratch whenever I felt the urge. Sometimes, I even felt guilty about it. At a doctor's appointment in the middle of that summer, my latest dermatologist actually told me not to scratch, to think of something else or do something else.

"Keep your hands busy. Try not to scratch them. Just ignore the itching," he had declared, as if it were the easiest thing on earth. I thought he must be from another planet. When my hands itched there was nothing on the face of the earth that would stop me from scratching them. Absolutely nothing could stop me from scratching the itch.

There was also a new problem. Over the summer, the itching had spread to a new body part, my feet. When it rained, I wore low, brown rubber boots that I put on over my shoes. They stopped at the ankle and were just high enough to keep my shoes dry. I started to get eczema where the rubber touched my ankles and even a little bit on the sides of my feet. Years later I would figure out that I was allergic to rubber, but it would take decades to realize this. And though this allergy was not the cause of my hand eczema, it would be revealed much later that coming into contact with rubber did cause my skin to itch. It was just one more annoyance. Itchy hands I could get used to, but feet were a lot harder to scratch.

KIDNAPPED

Chapter 5

THE LATE SUMMER day started like any other day – breakfast of eggs and toast in the kitchen nook and then outside to play in the warm August sun. Danny wasn't around so I walked the opposite way down the block toward Kathy's house. I didn't play too much with Kathy. She had lots of brothers and sisters and a big extended family that lived in other parts of town. She just wasn't around much. But that day seemed like a good day to see if maybe she was home.

I made it about halfway to Kathy's house when the trouble began. From both sides of the street the older neighborhood kids approached me. The leader was Mary's brother, who came up to me first. Behind him were Susan, Mary, and a guy I had never seen before. Barb was there too. I stopped dead in my tracks. Mary's brother spoke first.

"Your mother told us she had to go somewhere, and she asked us to take you over to Mrs. O'Donnell's house."

Mrs. O'Donnell lived clear around the block and I had visited her once or twice while riding bikes with Danny. But that was it. I did not really know her very well and my mother would never have me stay with her while she "went somewhere." I had never even had a babysitter. My mother did not believe in that. If she could not be home for some reason, then I would stay with one of my aunts. And never in a million years would my mother ask these neighborhood hoodlums to walk me somewhere! The whole thing was another big fat lie. They were coming toward me, arms outstretched. The guy I had never seen before took one of my arms and Mary's brother took the other. The girls formed a circle around me. I was trapped.

"Let me go!" I shouted.

"But your mother told us to take you around the block," came the quick reply.

"She did not!" I shot back. "That's a lie. She would never do that."

"Yes, she asked us to take you," and with that they pulled me down the sidewalk toward the end of the street. I fought with every inch of my body, twisting and turning out of their grip and yelling at the top of my lungs.

"Let me go!" I may have been shy, but I was not a pushover. Mary's brother tightened his grasp on my arm, but I was too much for him. I broke free and ran for home, breathless but safe.

What terrors awaited me around that corner I would never know. I may not have made it to Kathy's house, but what I learned that day was far more valuable. I was stronger than I thought. I had a voice and for the first time, despite my shyness, I had used it. I could stick up for myself when it counted. Their little plan had not worked. I had outsmarted five of them, fought back, and won, not quite realizing at the time just how much my newly discovered strength and voice would be needed in the years to come.

IS IT GOING TO HURT?

Chapter 6

"IS IT GOING to hurt?" I asked. I was standing near a giant, steel machine in yet another doctor's office in downtown Schenectady, New York. A few weeks into the new school year, after settling into my fourth-grade classroom, my parents decided that I needed to see an out-of-town dermatologist for the eczema. After multiple visits with the local Gloversville doctors, the eczema was no better. My father asked around town for some good dermatologists "down the line," as Schenectady and the capital city of Albany were called. To get a second opinion we needed to travel, so we made the hour-long drive to Schenectady, hopeful that a big city doctor would promise a cure.

I was terrified of doctors and any kind of medical procedure. I was still quite shy, but not when confronted with some unknown treatment or piece of equipment. Again, my timid nature vanished as I proclaimed my apprehensions loudly and clearly. The doctor chuckled, my parents chuckled, and I found no humor in it at all.

"No," he replied. "It is not going to hurt. It is just like an x-ray machine taking a picture."

I still hesitated. The doctor stopped smiling and seemed a bit agitated. I didn't like him.

The contraption was dark gray, ominously rising all the way up to the ceiling. And adding to my anxiety, another suspicious thought was forming. A machine was going to make my eczema go away? It seemed too easy. And why had no one else used this machine or even suggested it?

The doctor himself did not appear confident. He just wanted the procedure over with and me out of his office. I could not run out of there, although the thought crossed my mind. The doctor told me to put my hands inside the center of the steely machine. I did not trust him, but had no choice. Reluctantly, I placed my tiny, pale, shaking hands exactly where he told me to, always the dutiful child. And then the machine started, emitting some loud noises which I also did not like. But the doctor was right on one count – it didn't hurt. I was told to leave my hands in place and turn them palms up, then palms down. Although it felt like a long time, it was probably only a few seconds. I was relieved when it was over. I looked at my hands. They did not look any different. They just felt dry. The doctor handed my mother another prescription for steroid cream with the same directions as all the other steroid creams:

"Apply once in the morning and once at night."

As my dad completed some paperwork, I bolted out of there and ran to the car. I had survived the special machine but knew in my gut that my skin would be no better. And I was right.

Decades later, I would find out that I had been the recipient of high-dose radiation known as medical radiation. This procedure had been used since the 1920s to treat over eighty skin conditions. Eczema, psoriasis, and even acne sufferers were given these treatments on a regular basis, until excess radiation was linked with cancer. Fortunately, I only received the one treatment. We did not go back to Schenectady for a while – at least not for me.

UP IN SMOKE

Chapter 7

MY FATHER STARTED smoking in college. It was trendy and cool back then. Everybody smoked.

After college his habit grew to a pack a day, sometimes more. In the sixties, my father's job took him on the road during the week, which in one small way may have been a good thing. Research showed that secondhand smoke could contribute to eczema in children.

I always looked forward to the weekend, when my father came home. Each Friday evening, when I heard him climbing the stairs, I ran into the kitchen, jumped into his arms, and peeked to see what he had brought me. He always had a present for me. The best one was a pink truck that housed a dog kennel with twelve plastic dogs residing in separate kennels on the flatbed of the truck. A beagle, a collie, a dachshund – they were all there – the perfect gift for a little girl who loved dogs.

I loved to sit on the floor next to his chair as he read the newspaper and smoked. On one occasion, I reached up to try one of his cigarettes and pulled one out of the pack. He quickly took it out of my hand and told me I was too young, that cigarettes were for adults only. Still curious, I could have sneaked one at some point, but even as a young child I always followed the rules. I was obedient, people-pleasing, and conscientious, traits I would carry into adulthood.

The lung cancer began when my father was in his forties. The trips down the line were then for him, to Schenectady and Albany for cobalt treatments, a form of radiation used in the 1950s and '60s to treat some cancers. I have often wondered if there was a link between the onset and chronic nature of my eczema and the stress that I felt watching my father's struggle with cancer.

In June of 1965, my father bought a house for us, a cozy white bungalow with aqua shutters, in a cute neighborhood even closer to my elementary school. So we moved again. He must have wanted my mother and me to have a better place to live than a drafty old rented apartment. He always had a present for me, but this new home would turn out to be a bittersweet parting gift.

My father died on August 29, 1965, two months after my tenth birthday.

This date would have additional meaning for me in the future, but at the time, it ushered in the start of many changes in my life. Losing my father at such a young age left its mark on me in ways I would not fully realize until I was older.

MALENA MAN

Chapter 8

AS MY MOTHER and I adjusted to life without my father, our new home in the new neighborhood with all new friends provided a flicker of hope. I felt grateful that the taunting from the kids in the old neighborhood had become a thing of the past.

The backyard was huge, and in the center stood a catalpa tree, perfect for climbing. There was an enclosed back porch where I could play with my newfound friends. My mother loved it too. The bright, sunny kitchen sported new appliances, and we even had a washer and dryer. Like in the old apartment, there was a cozy kitchen nook, but this one had benches with bright red cushions, a window overlooking the backyard, and a light above the table shaped like a lantern. Mom hung a thermometer on the window, where each morning at breakfast we checked the temperature and talked about our daily plan.

One bright day that fall, I was home from school with a bad cold. I glanced around my beautiful new bedroom with pale pink walls, dainty white curtains, and a flower-print bedspread. Despite the cheerful sunlight pouring through my bedroom window, a feeling of sadness crept in. In only two months' time, I had lost my father, moved to a new neighborhood, and started a new school year with a new teacher. I had adapted to these changes with resilience, but the one thing that I hoped would change did not. I still had eczema. It followed me to the new house and showed no signs of leaving. In fact, it seemed quite pleased to settle in, appear, disappear, and reappear whenever the mood struck.

For two years, both my father and mother had hoped to find a cure for my problem skin and would have done anything to eradicate my eczema. The many trips to multiple doctors were proof of that. My father had always been supportive as he tried to help me deal with the eczema. He even accompanied me to one of my dermatologist's appointments despite not feeling well. Going forward though, the burden of my skin condition would become my mother's alone. She would be the only one watching me scratch my hands until they bled, and listening to my complaints about the nonstop itching while silently praying for a cure.

I soon realized that I would have to be strong, if not for myself then for my mother. I did not want my eczema to be another burden to her. She had lost her beloved husband and was struggling to move on. The new house was wonderful and provided a nice diversion, but my father's death had created a huge void that would not be easily filled. The last thing my mother needed was to hear me complain about my itchy hands. So on that sick day off from school, I tried to put a positive spin on my eczema situation.

I sat upright in my bed and eyed the latest treatment sitting on the nightstand, a flat metal tin of Malena ointment. A family friend had suggested it, saying it might possibly help the eczema. Malena was an older remedy, nonprescription and very mild, used since the mid-1900s for burns, blisters, and general skin irritations. It looked different from my other creams and ointments. I had been using it for two weeks, and was happy that it did not sting and actually felt somewhat soothing.

I grabbed the Malena tin and carefully positioned it in the center of a sheet of lined notebook paper, tracing around the tin to make a nice, even circle. I drew a head at the top, legs on the bottom, and arms out to the sides. I colored the circle with light-brown crayon to look like the tin and carefully wrote Ma-le-na across the circle. And just like that, "Malena Man" was created, the coolest of all paper dolls. I took scissors and meticulously cut him out, giving him life. Malena Man needed clothes, so I made him several outfits, including pajamas and a bathing suit. I showed him to my mother, who liked him very much. I had quietly hoped he would give her a chuckle, and Malena Man did not disappoint.

At ten years of age, I had instinctively conducted my own medical play therapy, unknowingly participating in my treatment. Years later I would learn that the process of imagining and creating Malena Man was a type of play therapy called "Child Life Therapy," a successful intervention widely used in hospitals to assist children in dealing with illness or injury. Of course, at the time, I had no idea that Malena Man was helping me develop healthy coping skills and perseverance.

Malena Man kept me company long enough for me to realize that he was about the only good thing that the Malena tin had provided. After rubbing the greasy ointment on my hands for nearly one month, the eczema was no better. Malena Man eventually retired to my desk. The tin was deposited into a dresser drawer to befriend the various tubes of steroid creams, until it began to smell funny and got tossed out.

THE MAD SCIENTIST

Chapter 9

DR. TOM, WITH his white hair, skinny frame, and rumpled appearance, looked much like Doc from "Back to the Future," and was the latest addition to my mother's arsenal of potential eczema cures. After two or three years seeing the same dermatologist, without any improvement in the eczema, my mother felt a change was needed. Hearing about Dr. Tom, she scheduled an appointment for me in January of 1969. His office, above a store in downtown Gloversville, resembled something out of an old movie. There wasn't much furniture in the office to begin with, and what was there looked like it had seen better days – a few cabinets with some old bottles and a rickety chair in the middle of the room where I was told to sit. It creaked to one side as I plopped myself onto it.

The new doctor wheeled up to me on an old stool with a confidence that belied his appearance. He was sure he could cure my eczema, and for a moment I believed him. My mother's face glowed with hope as she clung to every word he spoke. After looking at my hands he immediately ordered a blood test, based on his belief that eczema was caused by a problem in the blood. That actually made some sense to me. Maybe the mad scientist was onto something.

There was one problem – although a teenager by then and having been pretty healthy for most of my life, I was still somewhat squeamish and wary of any medical procedure. I was just not accustomed to being poked with a needle. In fact, I downright hated the idea and voiced it loudly and clearly. "Isn't there any other way or any other test that could be used?"

Dr. Tom ignored my question, so my mother calmly replied, "You have to do this."

I worried about the test for a few more minutes, but the hope that this might be the answer to my problem slightly reduced my anxiety about the needle stick. I got the blood drawn the next morning.

One week later, I anxiously climbed the steps to Dr. Tom's office. I had survived the blood test and was excited and more than ready to hear the results. I wondered what he would find in my blood that had caused all the itching for the last six years.

Dr. Tom suddenly appeared at the door of his office, like a superhero, minus a cape. "I have the results of your blood test," he proudly announced as he held up the paperwork in front of me.

"Your eczema is caused by high cholesterol."

I was fourteen years old and my cholesterol was 220.

"It is way too high and must be lowered by this special diet!" he commanded.

In 1969, few children ever had their cholesterol level tested. Ironically, not only had mine been tested, but apparently was the cause of my eczema.

On some level, I hoped Dr. Tom was right and I would be cured. The fact that this doctor gave me such a simple yet unusual cause for my eczema gave me a weird sense of hope. But the bigger part of me sensed that he really might be a mad scientist. He seemed to have blamed any blood test not in the normal range for whatever problem the patient had, a kind of lopsided cause and effect.

On the off chance that he was right, I started a strict low cholesterol diet the very next day. The biggest change was that I could no longer have eggs every day for breakfast. That would prove to be a challenge, since I had eaten one egg and a piece of buttered toast every morning since kindergarten. I missed my usual breakfast, but mostly I missed cheese! My love for it had started early and never waned. When I was three, I downed an entire bowl of cottage cheese that was meant for my father, mother, and me, while mom prepared the rest of the meal with her back turned. Cheese was difficult to give up, but I knew I needed to give the special diet my best shot. My mother supported the endeavor by preparing both the appropriate foods and other foods that I liked, and encouraged me to see it through.

At first, she seemed optimistic that this new diet would improve my skin and was definitely worth a try. But despite her outwardly upbeat attitude, and all her efforts to please me in the process, we both silently wondered whether this cholesterol-lowering meal plan would be the answer to my eczema problem.

After two months of deprivation, I was sent for another blood test. My cholesterol level had indeed improved, but sadly my eczema had not. Dr. Tom really had no explanation for this. We left his office disappointed once again by the world of doctors. My mother's face showed her frustration and I felt bad for her also. In some ways she was suffering as much as I with the lack of improvement in my skin. Our faith in the medical profession, specifically dermatologists, had been declining. When I was first diagnosed with eczema and not cured by the prescribed steroid cream, we had doubts about that particular doctor's ability. But after six years of visiting multiple specialists offering a variety of treatments, my mother and I began to question what was really going on. Did anyone have any real answers?

Needless to say, we did not go back to the mad scientist and I filed away the experience as just another failure. On the bright side, I eagerly began to eat eggs and cheese again.

KEY-BORED

Chapter 10

MY MOTHER COULD type ninety words a minute at her job as a secretary in the Gloversville school system. She had been the fastest and most accurate typist in her business school classes, and that typing speed only increased when she began working. She took great pride in her keyboard abilities.

I decided to take a required typing class during the summer before my sophomore year of high school. A summer school typing class would give me something fun to do and hopefully alleviate the occasional boredom of summer vacation. Hearing the loud click-clack of the keys as my mother typed recipes on our old typewriter only solidified my desire to learn this skill. I never gave my eczema a thought, or its potential effects on learning a mechanical skill like typing. In fact, I was trying to ignore it as much as possible ever since the special diet from the mad scientist had failed so miserably. I was taking a break from doctors, and the typing class would be a great diversion.

The class was held three days a week for six weeks. The first day of class went well. We met our teacher, Mr. Johnson, who had a great personality, joked with us, and seemed happy to be teaching on a beautiful summer day. We repeatedly hit the same keys over and over and were told to practice at home. We typed some simple words and learned not to ever look at the keys. I followed very carefully and promised myself that I would never look. I knew I could be as fast on the keyboard as my mother!

When I got home the first day, I practiced for a couple of minutes until the phone rang. My friend Julie wanted to ride bikes. That suddenly sounded a whole lot better than practicing typing indoors. "Well, I did practice a little," I reasoned as I headed out the door. The next day in class it was apparent that some of the kids had practiced for more than a few minutes. I could hear their keystrokes going faster than mine. We quickly reviewed the prior day's lesson and then were on to new letters and new words. I already felt the need to catch up. I told myself that I would practice more. But on that second evening, I did not feel like it. It was not as much fun as I thought it would be. I also realized something else – my eczema, which seemed to have gotten worse, made pressing on the typewriter keys uncomfortable . The skin on my right thumb was cracked, and bled a little as I repeatedly hit the spacebar. Reaching up to pound the letter P with my pinky finger did not feel too great either. The big lesson I learned that day was that typing and hand eczema were not a good match.

The third day we were given a pop quiz. I struggled to complete it and received a C. I glanced around the room and saw a few Bs and a couple of As. It was only the first week of class and I was already behind. I vowed to practice more, but each evening the same thing happened. I just didn't want to. The weekend was no better. That was not how I had expected the summer to go.

Week two of class began with learning more letters and typing small sentences. On a second pop quiz I received a D. I had never gotten a D in my life. I was mortified. I was the worst student in the class. When I reluctantly told my mother, she advised me to practice more, but I was already so far behind, hated practicing, and worst of all, my hands hurt with every strike of the keys. I wanted to be outside with friends in the summer, not inside pounding my itchy hands on an old typewriter.

The situation only got worse. I was in a class with overachievers. They were flying over the keys, acing the quizzes and giving me looks of pity. "Poor Claire, she is just not getting it."

I began to feel sorry for myself and regretted taking a class in the summer. Overriding these thoughts was the unpleasant realization that I was about to be an embarrassment to my mother. She was the world's greatest typist and her only child was failing typing class!

As bad as I felt about the mess I was in, I could not bring myself to practice more. The class was almost over and it was simply too late to improve. I had secured my position as the worst student in the class. The Cs and Ds had turned into Fs. My only hope was somehow doing well on the final exam. I tried to think positive and actually practiced for a few minutes the night before.

On the morning of the test, I felt extremely nervous as I took my seat at the typewriter. I glared at it, hating its cold, threatening presence. I prayed for a miracle – some sudden strength of hands and fingers, agility, speed, and accuracy. I hoped my typing would not be interrupted by itchy hands. Muddling through the exam, with only one quick scratch, I knew I had made a few mistakes. But I kept going to complete everything before the time limit.

When the test was finally over, I felt relieved and glad I did not have to go to any more classes. I was hopeful for at least a passing grade, even though I didn't deserve it. Perhaps the teacher had taken pity on me and my eczematous hands. In reality, I was not sure that he actually knew about the eczema. I just assumed that he could see it. A few days later the results arrived in the mail. Luckily, I was alone in the house as I opened the envelope. A big, fat F stared back at me. In fact, there were two Fs – one on the final exam and one for the final grade. It was official. I had failed a class for the first time in my life.

I was ashamed of the grade, and dreaded telling my mother. I gave her the news the second she arrived home from work – the place where she typed all day, really fast, really well, spectacularly well.

"What do you mean, you failed?" she asked as her eyes darted around the room like fireflies on steroids.

"I failed the final exam and the class," I murmured.

"You didn't practice enough! You did not take the class seriously. You should have practiced more!"

"My hands hurt when I type," I countered. "The eczema bothers me when I hit the keys!"

Her anger softened a bit, but I still felt awful. I had disappointed her and that was extremely upsetting to me. But there was also another problem. Since typing was a required class at Gloversville High School, I would have to retake the class to graduate.

The next day, my mother's anger had subsided. She actually started to feel bad for me. She realized the cracked and bloody, itchy hands were at least partly to blame. She called the school and tried to get the F grade removed from my permanent record. She talked about the eczema and how difficult it was to practice with all the itching and scratching going on. It sounded like the person at the other end was sympathetic. My mother hung up the phone looking relieved. I too felt much better. I appreciated the fact that she had gone to bat for me. Her actions inspired me to advocate for myself in the future, a skill that would surely be needed.

A full year later I retook the class and got a B, same teacher and all. Some leftover typing experience from the first class, as well as more practice, helped, despite my itchy hands. I learned that failure did not have to be permanent. With resilience and determination, I could succeed.

BADGE OF HONOR

Chapter 11

IN HIGH SCHOOL, I did not date much at first. Eczema actually had nothing to do with it. Losing my father at an early age and having no brothers caused me to be a bit uncomfortable with guys. I was not used to being around them and did not know how to start a conversation. On the other hand, I met some very nice girlfriends who filled the dating void. We rode bikes, took long walks, and went out for pizza. We also went to the high school dances, where I mostly stood on the side or danced with guys who were merely friends. I had not cracked the high school code of popularity just yet.

In my sophomore year I tried out to be a baton twirler in the Gloversville High School band, which performed during fall football games and in parades. Autumn in upstate New York could be cold and windy, and baton twirlers could not wear gloves. Determined to make this forty-person squad, I was not about to let eczema and dry, cracked hands stop me. I was ecstatic when I was selected and received the cute uniform. The twirlers wore a white sweater with a large maroon chenille "G" on the front. Our pleated skirts were maroon, with white inside the pleats, which popped out when we marched. We sported high white boots adorned with maroon pom-poms made from yarn. I was a twirler for two years and loved it. But there was something even better on the horizon.

I really wanted to be a Shakerette. In the hierarchy of high school activities, this was at the top. Only a dozen girls were chosen for the squad. The Shakerettes were dancers, carrying huge white pom-poms made out of white netting. With high kicks, they marched onto the football field first and stood in front of the twirlers. They were the elite group of the high school marching band. I longed to be a part of it.

I had auditioned to be a Shakerette for my junior year, but was not selected. I had not memorized the dance well enough. I was still a twirler, so all was not lost, but I vowed to audition again the following year. I practiced, memorized, and performed the routine flawlessly, and was not surprised when I made the squad for my senior year. I hoped this would help my popularity. I traded in my white sweater and maroon skirt for the opposite colors – a maroon sweater with a white chenille "G" on the front and a white skirt with maroon in the pleats. I put my baton in the closet and hugged my gigantic new pom-poms. I had arrived. I loved the dancing even more than the twirling. Shaking pom-poms did not hurt as much as twirling a baton, a big plus for my still itchy, scratchy hands. Shakerettes had a special march onto the football field, something the twirlers did not. I mastered it quickly, probably from having seen it so often. In prior years, I had watched with envy as the Shakerettes performed this sexy march, and I was finally getting to do it.

With all the fun activities in my senior year, I became slightly less shy, more comfortable around boys, and even had a few dates. No one ever noticed my hand eczema, or if they did, it was not mentioned. I never felt self-conscious or embarrassed, or tried to hide it. In fact, I even showed my partially scabbed-over thumb to one boy who commented that it was indeed kind of gross. But this did not affect his desire to date me. At the time, I did not know anyone with eczema, and in a way that alone made me feel special. I had lived with eczema for nine years and survived, even thrived. Despite my frustration with the frequent itching, I liked being unique. The eczema had actually become a trophy of my toughness, a badge of honor that made me seem strong for living with it.

DOUBLE TROUBLE

Chapter 12

I GRADUATED HIGH school in June of 1973 and left Gloversville to attend Siena College in Loudonville, New York, majoring in Sociology. A small, private college near Albany, Siena was only one hour's drive from Gloversville, perfect for my first time away from home. I liked that Siena was a Catholic college, as I was raised Catholic and regularly attended Mass. More importantly, Siena enrolled twice as many men as women. But despite the favorable odds, I did not date much that first year. College life was an adjustment, and I had my hands full getting used to living in a dormitory and taking classes that I found much harder than those in high school.

At the start of my second year at Siena, I met David, who became my first real boyfriend. Soon after, my eczema flared again, but this time not only on my hands. For the first time in my life, the eczema suddenly appeared on my scalp as well. Three days later, the scalp eczema migrated to my face. A dry, itchy patch appeared on my forehead and another on the side of my cheek. Again, no one really noticed but I started to become slightly self-conscious about my badge of honor. I did find it odd that the eczema could even survive there, since the rest of my face was so oily. Why didn't the oil cancel out the eczema? After all, my dermatologist was always telling me to moisturize, moisturize, moisturize. I already had a significant oil slick going on. Adding any more oil to the mix would surely have alerted Greenpeace.

I worried that the eczema on my face and scalp would permanently come and go, like the eczema on my hands. I had started to accept the hand eczema after dealing with it for eleven years, but my face and scalp were a whole different story. Eczema had always been a physical problem for me, with all the itching, bloody fingers, and sleep deprivation due to scratching. But the relocation to new body parts was affecting my mindset as well, so I found yet another new dermatologist for some help. Since I did not own a car, David drove me to my appointment in Albany.

The doctor, with dark hair and spectacles, looked like an older Harry Potter. I hoped he would work some magic on my skin.

"Hello there!" he said brightly. "What brings you in today?"

"I have eczema on my hands and now it has migrated to my face and scalp." I added, "I can live with it on my hands, but my face is…" I paused for a minute. "Please do something."

"I can give you a new steroid cream for the facial eczema and that should clear it up," he promised.

I liked his positive, upbeat attitude, and felt a brief moment of relief. What he said next was a different story.

"And I am prescribing a special product for you to use on your scalp. Coal tar shampoo."

What? Coal tar?

"You can use it instead of regular shampoo and that should clear up the scalp eczema." He sounded confident, but as usual I had my doubts. After all, I had used dozens of skin creams, lotions, and ointments with zero success. Would this time be any different?

I left his office with more questions than answers. *What will the shampoo smell like? What if it doesn't work? What if the steroid cream doesn't clear up my facial eczema?*

I had persevered with all my previous skin treatments, so as the always-obedient patient, I would give the new prescriptions my best shot.

Back in the dorm, after waiting a few minutes until no one was around, I jumped quickly into the shower, armed with coal tar and ready to do battle with my scalp. The shampoo actually *did* look and smell like the tar used to pave highways. I worried that my hair would still smell of tar when I was done shampooing. And there was a gnawing feeling that if the treatment failed, I would be stuck with eczema on my scalp for all eternity. Nonetheless, I let the shampoo stay on for a few minutes, as the directions stated. Dutifully, I rinsed and repeated, feeling like a chia pet as my scalp seemed to move, flutter, and tingle.

Amazingly, the coal tar actually worked! Three shampoos and no smell later, the itching was completely gone and my scalp and hair were back to normal. On top of that, the new steroid cream worked like a charm and the eczema on my face disappeared as quickly as it had arrived. Harry Potter had worked his magic. I was overjoyed.

PIZZA AND STEROIDS

Chapter 13

IN THE SPRING of 1975, I neared the end of my sophomore year at Siena. Dormitory living had a highly positive impact on me, providing a camaraderie that I had never known before. Growing up as an only child, I sometimes felt isolated and alone. Residence hall life was the exact opposite. I took to the lively atmosphere in the dorm like pepperoni to pizza. There was always someone to hang out with or talk to. Late-night conversations were commonplace, about everything from classes, careers, or dating to the meaning of life.

Although still not self-conscious about it, by this time my hand eczema started to be more of an annoyance, and came more often than it went. The itching seemed to be increasing in both frequency and duration. In the past I had kept my struggles with eczema to myself, but the group living situation fortunately created a level of trust that allowed me to open up about my frustrations with it. One night in mid-April, I shared a late-night pizza with my dorm friends, one of whom happened to be a pre-med student. I felt comfortable enough with them to share my challenges with eczema. "I've had eczema on my hands since I was eight. It goes away sometimes but it always comes back. When it returns, I use steroid cream on it, but that doesn't always help," I revealed.

Ellen, the pre-med student and close friend, responded quickly, "Have you ever tried using the steroid cream every day, even when you don't have symptoms? Maybe if enough of the cream gets into your system, it will build up and the eczema will go away for good."

Ellen's idea made sense and I trusted her knowledge since she was a pre-med student. I began using the steroid cream twice a day for the rest of April and into early May. Each morning and night, I forced myself to rub the steroid cream on my hands. Using smelly, greasy cream that often was not pleasant, but I was determined to at least try her suggestion.

Ellen's advice, however, while well-intentioned, was incorrect. Some creams such as Elidel (Pimecrolimus) were later recommended for use on a daily or even twice-daily basis for up to four months to alleviate symptoms. But those creams were not available yet. Steroid creams, on the other hand, were not meant for long-term use. Most doctors prescribed steroids only to treat a flare-up of the disease, not for daily application, which Ellen was recommending. Of course, my twice-a-day ritual made no difference in my symptoms. The eczema still came and went, like an unwelcome houseguest, staying a few days, then finally leaving, only to return again a few days later. Ellen may have eventually gone on to medical school, but I stayed firmly planted in eczema hell.

SCENE CHANGE

Chapter 14

IN SEPTEMBER OF 1975, I transferred to the State University of New York at Plattsburgh, changing my major to elementary education, which Siena did not offer. My two-year program required both teaching courses and electives. Of all the electives to choose from I settled on a beginning piano class, thinking that playing the piano would fit well with an elementary teaching degree. I had always wanted to take piano lessons, and as a bonus I would receive college credit.

As luck would have it, our professor was actually a famous concert pianist, which made me even more excited to get started. We began to learn some basic skills, such as proper hand position and how to move the fingers to play scales. With all the beginners banging on the keys it was chaos for most of the semester, forcing our teacher to cover her ears and yell "Stop!" on several occasions.

I vowed to practice as much as I could. One evening, I found an old piano in one of the dorm lounges and forced myself to sit down and play. It was there that I had a flashback. This was typing class all over again! The teacher was continually telling me to bend my fingers over the keys, but the eczema on my hands prevented me from achieving the proper finger position. If I bent them correctly, they cracked and bled. Lotions and creams did not help. Like the keys on a piano, my situation was black and white. I had eczema and it hurt to play the piano.

Thirteen years of eczema torment with no end in sight, I thought to myself. Once again, the condition was affecting my daily life and making it difficult to do the things I wanted to do. I muddled through the remainder of the semester, attending every session and dutifully practicing as best I could. Even so, I began to worry about failing the class. As a college student I no longer had the advantage of having my mother advocate for me, as she had done with typing class. I finally told my professor that I had eczema and how it was affecting my playing, hoping for understanding when it came to my class grade. My theory worked. She suggested the pass-fail option so that the C grade that I actually earned would not lower my overall grade point average. I readily accepted her offer. Unlike typing class, at least I had passed this one, albeit by the skin of my teeth. Uh…fingers.

ഌ   ഌ   ഌ

Continuing to try new things by putting activities in the foreground and eczema in the background, I joined the Plattsburgh Dolphins Synchronized Swim Club in my second semester. I was already a good swimmer, but this type of swimming was completely different. I always enjoyed a challenge and was able to master a few underwater skills that involved holding my breath for an extended period of time. Swimming provided a nice diversion and took my mind off eczema. Being in the water actually made my hands feel better, and softened their roughness, if only for a short time. Although chlorine was known to make eczema worse in some people, it had no effect on others, as in my case. I certainly was not allergic to it, but the strong chlorine did not cure my skin either.

At the end of my first year at Plattsburgh, I was asked to participate in a synchronized swimming show for the campus. My proficiency had improved, and a performance would allow me to show off my new skills. I swam in a duet with my roommate and a group number with several of my teammates. I loved the fancy lighting and music being piped into the pool, but also noticed the small number of spectators in the stands. Synchronized swimming was not yet popular and it would be years before it became an Olympic sport. But I really did not care that the audience was small. I was just happy to participate in something new and unique. Eczema had not stopped me. In fact, eczema was the furthest thing from my mind as I held my breath and joined my teammates in the finale, a synchronized dive to the bottom of the pool. Popping back up to the surface, I heard the audience applaud and knew our show had been a success. Perhaps having new experiences, finding distractions, keeping busy, and staying positive were the real answers to living with eczema.

My success with synchronized swimming gave me a renewed sense of confidence. I could take on new challenges and succeed, despite living with a bothersome skin condition. *So what if typing and playing the piano aren't my thing?* There was a whole world out there with all kinds of other options. Transferring to Plattsburgh was a great decision. A myriad of clubs, sports, and other activities made this college extra fun.

In the fall of 1976, I entered my senior year at Plattsburgh. As I walked by the gym on my way to class one day, I stumbled upon Acro Théâtre, which I later discovered was actually gymnastics set to music and performed for an audience in a theatre setting. Through the doorway, I saw students flipping on giant mats, swinging from uneven bars, and bouncing on trampolines. That got my attention. I was mesmerized. Replaying the wonderful memories of jumping on the neighborhood trampoline as a child, I knew I had to join this group. Starting gymnastics at the advanced age of twenty-one would be difficult, but I was no stranger to challenges and at least I had the trampoline experience! I joined the Acro Théâtre club the next day, not giving eczema even a single thought.

I loved jumping on the trampoline again, and with a gymnastics coach present I was free to try new skills with little chance of injury. I learned both front and back flips and even attempted a back layout. The coach also taught floor exercise, uneven bars, balance beam, and vault. The bars, beam, and vault were difficult, and I was not able to do much. And although initially I did not think it would be an issue, the hand eczema made it uncomfortable to hang onto the uneven bars. Once, while dismounting from the bars, I miscalculated and landed flat on my back. I got the wind knocked out of me and fear knocked into me. That was pretty much the end of my quest to be the next great Olympic gymnast!

At the end of the year the Acro Théâtre club presented a gymnastics show for the campus. I performed in two numbers and my picture appeared in the university newspaper, which became the highlight of my gymnastics career. The performance was bittersweet. It marked the end of my gymnastics club days, as well as the end of college.

I never went to the dermatologist while in Plattsburgh. Eczema was still coming and going, like my coming and going to practices. If my eczema wasn't curable, learning to live with it was the next best thing. There was just too much to do – too many classes, activities, and good times to let eczema limit me. After all, when in life would I get to do all these neat, fun, and different things again, while at the same time putting eczema in the background? Plattsburgh would be the only city I ever lived in where I did not search for a skin doctor.

STRESS-CZEMA

Chapter 15

AFTER GRADUATION IN June 1977, I moved back home to Gloversville. I worked as a substitute teacher in several elementary schools until January 1978, when I was offered a temporary position replacing a teacher who was taking maternity leave through the rest of the school year. Although it was a wonderful opportunity to jump-start my career, the job presented a difficulty I had not foreseen. As a brand-new teacher just out of college, I did not have enough experience to properly take over the classroom in the middle of the year. The children were used to their regular teacher, who was excellent and had years of teaching experience. I struggled to gain control of the classroom. The challenge was greater than a back flip on the trampoline. Stress set in. And so did my eczema.

The transition from my carefree college days into the real world of work and teaching was not an easy one for me. I missed college, all my sporting activities at Plattsburgh, living in the dorm, and the friends I had made. After one month of teaching, my eczema returned with a vengeance, this time reappearing on my face and scalp. I made the trip down the line once more to yet another dermatologist who prescribed the usual remedies – steroid cream for my face and my old friend the coal tar shampoo for my hair, the stuff of highway pavement. Fortunately, the treatment still worked. But after fifteen years of dealing with the unpredictable nature of my eczema, it seemed there was no end in sight.

Teaching was taking its toll. The temporary job that was presumably paving the way to a permanent one was wreaking havoc on my skin and my health. I began to get headaches at the end of the workday that required an hour-long nap when I finally arrived home exhausted. I wondered if the eczema mirrored what was happening in my life. At times, both my classroom and my skin felt like a volcano about to erupt, as if the bubbling and itching of the eczema echoed the chaos I sometimes felt while trying to succeed at work with my limited skills. It was a long six months. Was this even what I was supposed to be doing? Neither the naps nor scratching helped. Was the itch of the eczema a reflection of an itch to do something different with my life?

When the school year finally ended in June, I looked forward to the summer break, free time, and warmer weather, which I hoped would lessen my eczema. The teacher I had replaced for six months would return in the fall and my temporary job would be over. Perhaps my next teaching job would be easier, with the benefit of six month's experience. At the time, however, there were more teachers than jobs for them, especially in our small town. So, with no job on the horizon, I had to come up with a Plan B. In the meantime I enjoyed the break, swimming, biking, and spending time with friends. Not surprisingly, with the stress of replacing an experienced teacher out of the picture, the eczema improved slightly and my headaches went completely away. A small voice was telling me that it might be time to pursue another career path. Perhaps eczema was a compass for direction in my life. If so, I had to follow it.

LANE CHANGE AHEAD

Chapter 16

WHEN THE NEW academic year began in fall of 1978, I resumed substitute teaching at various schools throughout the county. This was slightly less stressful, as I just filled in for a day or two. I knew I was only there temporarily. What was *not* temporary was my eczema. The intense itching had returned and was really bothering me. The cold autumn weather seemed to make the eczema worse and contributed to my misery. I scratched my hands constantly and gave up on the steroid cream. The fun synchronized swimming and gymnastics diversions I had enjoyed in college were not available for adults in Gloversville. Riddled with anxiety, the itch to do something else weighed on my mind and on my skin, but I didn't know where to turn.

I confided to my mother that I needed a different career path, possibly an alternative to teaching, since there were no jobs currently available. Substituting was enjoyable at times, but did not provide the benefits of full-time work. My mother was of course sympathetic, but unable to offer career guidance, so she did the next best thing by asking her boss, a high school principal, for ideas. He thought for a moment and said he had recently learned of an up-and-coming occupation called "industrial librarian." A master's degree in library science was needed to pursue this career route, and a librarian of this type would work in a business setting for a corporation. With a library degree, working in a school library would also be a possibility. My bachelor's degree in education was a great fit for this option. And just like that, with a perfect answer to my career woes, I jumped at the chance to pursue my Plan B.

I started immediately by asking to substitute for librarians and media specialists, instead of classroom teachers, in the county school system. I also began researching colleges that offered a Library Science program, and ultimately made the decision to go to graduate school in Florida. I wanted something different from the small-town atmosphere in Gloversville. While my hometown had been a wonderful place to grow up, I needed some more excitement. But mostly I hoped the warmer weather would improve my skin. Interestingly, as I concentrated on choosing a college and preparing for the GRE (Graduate Record Exam), a requirement to get into a master's program, my eczema faded into the background again. I was so focused on other tasks that I did not pay attention to it. I felt like I had regained control of my life. I applied and was accepted to the graduate program offered at the University of South Florida in Tampa. Sunshine and palm trees beckoned.

GOING THE DISTANCE

Chapter 17

LEAVING GLOVERSVILLE TO begin a new chapter of my life in Florida was filled with mixed emotions. I would miss my mother terribly and all my friends, but at twenty-three I knew it was something I had to do. I arrived in Tampa on January 2, 1979, one week before my graduate classes began. Since I was a new student, I needed some extra time to move into the residence hall and get settled, but hardly anyone was around yet. I felt lonely, and wondered if I had made a mistake. I also found an unwelcome surprise in my dormitory – roaches. I had never seen them before, and they seemed to be everywhere. I got home one evening and a small roach was sitting proudly on top of my hairbrush waving its antennae at me. I looked for another place to live, but roaches were commonplace in Florida, so my search for another dorm proved fruitless.

Eventually, the campus came alive with more than insects. I made new friends every day, lounged by the pool, attended parties, and biked to class. A month went by and I was starting to love Florida. I also loved my classes. It was such a relief to be majoring in Library Science, a field that felt like a good fit for me. The classes were interesting, the instructors enthusiastic and excited to be there. One professor talked of job opportunities after graduation. She spoke glowingly of careers in "special libraries," which I realized was the same as the industrial libraries that the high school principal had mentioned. The salaries were great, and the librarian was to be an integral part of the employee team and expected to be loyal to the company. It all sounded wonderful and reinforced my desire to go the special libraries route. The shyness of my youth had lessened somewhat, but my personality was still on the quiet side, so library work seemed to be a good fit in that respect also.

My days at the University of South Florida were some of the happiest of my life. Ironically, the eczema was no better in the Florida heat. It had followed me like a criminal's rap sheet. I could run, but I could not hide. I quickly discovered than sunny, happy days did not equate to happy skin. Years later I would come across an article in the *Journal of Investigative Dermatology* that warned, "Warm, humid, and high sun exposure climates are associated with poorly controlled eczema..." which explained my eczema's lack of improvement in Florida. Running off to Florida to escape eczema had been a futile mission.

BOOKS, BUCS, AND BEGINNINGS

Chapter 18

DESPITE THE LACK of improvement of my eczema in Florida, I was still happy that I had moved there. During my last quarter of graduate school in 1980, I looked forward to finding a job utilizing my new library science degree. The high school principal's suggestion to become a corporate librarian had proved to be a good one, and I was eager to see it through. With graduation on the horizon, I knew that my post-graduate college experience, with its many activities, friendships, and good times, would also be ending. I did not want a repeat of the sadness I felt when graduating from Plattsburgh with my bachelor's degree, so I hoped to replace some of the college fun and camaraderie with a new adventure. At the last minute I decided to audition for the Tampa Bay Buccaneers cheerleading squad, which performed at football games in Tampa Stadium. If I made it, I would also have the opportunity to relive my beloved high school Shakerettes days.

I made the first cut and was scheduled for final tryouts. Unfortunately, in the week prior, I caught the flu, my boyfriend broke up with me, and my car broke down. It was a terrible week. I forced myself to go to the rehearsals, but felt so sick that I sat on the bleachers and just watched as the other girls practiced the dance routine. Marching steps similar to the Shakerettes moves had been added, and I knew that if I had been able to practice, I would have mastered them. I actually tried out anyway, but not having properly learned the choreography, of course I did not make it. I chalked it all up to bad timing and marked my calendar for tryouts the following year.

The bright spot of the audition experience was lining up a great part-time job for the fall football season, as a press box hostess for the Tampa Bay Buccaneers. Handing out programs and statistics sheets and serving refreshments would keep me involved with a professional sports team, and would fit right in with the full-time corporate librarian job I was hoping to get. Things already looked promising and graduation was just around the corner.

With my master's degree in hand, I was ready for my close-up. But for a time, I had to be content with filling out job applications and working as a waitress to pay the bills. Finally, in August 1980, I landed my first library job at SmithKline Laboratories. It was a perfect entry-level position and would give me much-needed experience in my new career. As the librarian for the largest clinical laboratory in town, I ordered medical books and articles for the physicians and staff, and performed miscellaneous tasks such as covering the company's store a few hours a week. The job was not particularly stressful and suited my quiet personality. Best of all, I enjoyed going to work every day. I breathed a prayer of thanks to my mother and the high school principal for pointing me in the right direction.

TIME TO GET ROWDY

Chapter 19

MOVING TO FLORIDA had been a good decision, but the Sunshine State had certainly disappointed on one count – the eczema still plagued me. While it continued to do its usual dance of coming and going, mostly I ignored it, counting my blessings in other ways. A year after getting my first library job, I still liked it. I also enjoyed my press box hostess side hustle with the Tampa Bay Buccaneers, and life seemed to be going well. Although the calendar had reminded me, I did not audition again to be a Bucs cheerleader, perhaps a bit wary. But when the local newspaper announced cheerleading tryouts for another professional sports team in Tampa, I decided to give it a go. In September 1981, I auditioned for the Wowdies, the cheerleaders for the Tampa Bay Rowdies soccer team. Members of the North American Soccer League (NASL), the Rowdies were one of two professional sports teams in Tampa at the time.

I had been to a soccer game once and admired the cheerleaders dancing on the sidelines wearing green and white uniforms and holding sparkling pom-poms. So, at 7:00 on a Friday evening, I found myself entering a Tampa dance studio to audition once again to become a professional cheerleader. After filling out an application and pinning a number on my shirt, I discovered that this audition would be very different from the Bucs audition. The choreographer demonstrated a few dance steps and we practiced for a minute or two. Then, in groups of four, we performed the combination in front of the judges. With no chance to really memorize the steps, the audition became more of a test of will than anything. I did my best, but had a flashback to the Bucs audition and sensed that I might not make this squad either. Soon though, I realized something important. Several others were struggling too. I decided to try to look good doing the moves even if I did not do them exactly right. I kicked my right leg when I probably should have been kicking my left, but I kicked high and straight and smiled confidently. It seemed to get a little easier, and I noticed a couple of the judges looking at me and writing on their notepads. One even smiled back at me. Things were looking up. I left the audition feeling more hopeful than when I started.

Three days later I received a letter in the mail from the Tampa Bay Rowdies, the return address emblazoned with bold green letters. I ripped it open and learned I had made the first cut. I was to return to the studio in one week on another Friday evening for final auditions. This round required competing with the veteran Wowdies from the prior year. I was thrilled.

The evening of the audition, I planned my outfit carefully and took extra time getting ready. Because I was one of the first to arrive at the studio, I received a low number, indicating that I would be in one of the first groups to perform before the judges. But it also meant less time to learn the combination. As I thought about this concern, I watched the veteran dancers enter the studio, wearing the Wowdies practice uniform, a blue leotard with pale pink tights. Those with long hair wore it up in a tight bun. The girls exuded confidence and were absolutely beautiful. I immediately felt intimidated. I would compete not just with experienced dancers, but with a group of girls who looked like models.

Without much fanfare, the choreographer walked to the front of the room and began to demonstrate the steps for the audition. Every eye was focused on her. My nerves took a back seat as I concentrated on memorizing the steps. I was in the second group of four to go before the judges; this would turn out to be a good thing. I would get it over with quickly, so nervousness would not have time to get a strong hold on me. "Learn it, act like I know it, project confidence, and dance it out!" I told myself.

The first combination was pretty simple and I thought I had it down. Smiling as brightly as I could, I strutted to the center of the room and tried to follow my own advice. A minute later it was over and I felt good about my efforts. I watched as the other groups came forward. The veteran dancers were fabulous. They did every step perfectly and were cool, calm, and confident, almost to the point of arrogance. I so wanted to be one of them.

We were quickly taught another short dance, this one quite a bit harder. I would have to fake it a bit, as I did not get a couple of the steps. "Look confident," I repeated to myself. I practiced in the back for another moment and then it was my turn again. I had heard that with auditions of this type, showing potential would be the biggest factor in making the squad.

"Just keep going!" I reminded myself when I realized I was on the wrong foot. "The judges don't always know the exact steps; they're just looking for promise." Another minute later it was over, and I still felt good about my efforts.

After several more combinations performed in the same groups, the choreographer told us we had one final thing to do. We were to move diagonally across the floor in front of the judges, one at a time, doing any dance steps we wanted. This was perfect for me, as I always enjoyed improvising. It was not the time to be invisible, so I dug deep to dredge up some old Shakerettes steps, overcame my nerves, and boldly danced across the floor. I made it up as I went along, smiling and making eye contact with each of the judges. It was over before I knew it, and I felt optimistic. Next, I just had to wait for the results.

The letter arrived three days later, on Monday, September 21, 1981, to be exact. Tearing it open, I immediately saw the word "Congratulations" at the top of the letter. I was so excited I could hardly stand it. "You have been selected as a 1981–1982 Tampa Bay

Wowdie. We hope you will find the coming year to be an exciting one. As a new Wowdie, you have become part of a group that is highly esteemed not only for its dance activities but also for its community involvement. Rehearsals begin Tuesday, September 29, from 8:30 to 10:00 p.m." I could hardly wait for Tuesday to arrive to start this new adventure.

My dream to be a professional cheerleader had come true. The Rowdies soccer team was attracting a lot of attention, and the stadium often filled up with twenty thousand fans on game nights. I would get to relive my Shakerettes days after all, cheer for a professional sports team, and build camaraderie with a new group of friends. My self-confidence was at an all-time high. And once again, eczema was the furthest thing from my mind.

DANCE-OFF

Chapter 20

AT THE FIRST rehearsal, before dancing a single step, we were introduced to our director, choreographer, and teachers, and reviewed the Wowdie regulations that we were expected to follow during the season. The Rowdies played indoor soccer from December through mid-February, and after a short break, outdoor soccer began at Tampa Stadium and continued through the summer. Wowdies' rehearsals were scheduled every Tuesday and Thursday from 8 to 10 p.m. at the studio, and on the stadium field before each game. All practices and home games were mandatory, with three excused absences allowed per season. A fourth or any unexcused absence resulted in automatic dismissal. During the year the cheerleaders were required to represent the Rowdies franchise with a minimum of five appearances in uniform at pep rallies, store openings, festivals, and local events. At first glance this endeavor appeared to be quite time-consuming, but I was ready to commit. It was time to dance.

As our choreographer began teaching the first combination, I received a rude awakening. She demonstrated it only once, and then it was our turn. I soon realized that this would be more challenging than I had ever imagined. Besides Shakerettes, my dance background consisted of a few months of ballet and tap when I was eleven and a handful of beginning ballet and jazz classes while I was in college. So to say that I was not adequately prepared for what was to come was an understatement. I looked around the room and noticed that many of the girls, the veterans, had the sequence down right away. There were also a few girls, some of the newly selected Wowdies, who looked like deer in the headlights. I was one of them.

As the night wore on, we struggled. Our teacher, sensing this, began to break down some of the steps, making them easier to learn. This helped a little, but I was finding it hard to remember what came next. I would get the first two or three parts but when it was all put together, I just could not remember them. I tried following the people around me, but this strategy caused me to often be a count or two behind the rest of the group. At times, it was almost like two separate dances going on – one all perfectly choreographed and executed and the other all messy and disconnected. At least I was not alone in my discomfort.

When the first rehearsal finally ended, I realized two things. Most importantly, despite my first-night jitters and difficulties, I loved the experience. But I also knew, without a doubt, that I would need to tap into my resilience and perseverance to properly learn both the choreographer's style and the dance steps in order to succeed. At our second rehearsal, it was more of the same – stressful but admittedly still fun. Near the end of that evening, I chatted with some of the veteran Wowdies and was relieved to discover that many of them had taken years of dance classes from a very young age. My limited dance background could not compare to their extensive experience. It was as simple as that.

After a few weeks of rehearsals, a second choreographer was brought in to assist with teaching and to help select the group of cheerleaders who would perform the halftime show at the indoor opening game. Everyone would be allowed to dance on the sidelines, but the main dance performance in the center of the arena would be limited to only those dancers who passed an audition. I knew I would not make it. In fact, I was secretly hoping that I would not be selected so that I could learn the ropes from the sidelines at the first game. The halftime audition was held two weeks prior to the highly anticipated season opener with the Montreal Manics. As expected, I did not make it. There were several of us who would stand on the sideline and watch as the others performed in the center of the arena during the break in the soccer action. It was totally okay with me to be in the group *not* chosen. I knew all the sideline dances well and would be able to just take it all in without the anxiety of performing during halftime. I could hardly wait.

My first game as a Rowdies cheerleader was awesome in every way. It was held indoors at the Bayfront Center in St. Petersburg on December 5, 1981. I loved the Wowdies' new uniforms, white satin jackets with the Rowdies logo embroidered in green letters on the front, white and green striped shorts, and sneakers with a green stripe down the side. The Tampa Bay Rowdies organization always offered wonderful promotions at their games for their Fannies, as their fans were called. As Wowdies, we were often asked to participate. That night we handed out free drink cups and champagne to the first five thousand Fannies entering the stadium. After chatting with a few fans, it quickly became crowded and hectic and it was all I could do to make sure each person received a cup. Noting the growing numbers, it sank in that I would be performing in front of 7,500 fans that filled the Bayfront Center to capacity. I began to feel nervous until I remembered that I would be dancing *only* on the sidelines that evening. Ultimately, it was an exciting first night as a Wowdie, and we all had a blast dancing on the sidelines, half watching the game and half anticipating our next dance steps. I would have the luxury of easing into that halftime spotlight with more experience. In the meantime, I was just thrilled to be a member of the Tampa Bay Rowdies professional sports organization.

ITCHY POMS

Chapter 21

AFTER THREE MONTHS of rehearsals, I grew more accustomed to the dance style and the moves were easier to learn. I became friends with another dancer who helped me catch on to some of the more difficult steps. We finished the indoor season at the end of February and began preparing for the outdoor soccer games that would take place in front of an even bigger crowd at Tampa Stadium.

I received a different uniform for the outdoor season – a short dress with a white top and green skirt. Once again, the Wowdies logo was embroidered across the front, this time in even larger letters. I loved it. But my favorite addition to the new uniform was the big, fluffy, green and white pom-poms, which we had not used during the indoor season. Like the ones I used as a Shakerette, they were so much fun to dance with and made me really feel like a professional cheerleader.

The Rowdies' home opener vs. Tulsa Roughnecks played to twenty thousand excited Fannies on April 3, 1982. Television cameras and media were everywhere. By that point, all of us had significantly improved and performed together in the halftime show in the center of the stadium. I knew the dance well and was able to pull it off, despite a huge case of nerves. Back on the sidelines, and out of the direct spotlight, I still enjoyed the quick, easy sideline dances that were well memorized. I even relaxed enough to look around and revel in the exciting atmosphere of the first match of the Rowdies' outdoor season – until I had an unexpected visitor. My right hand began to itch…a lot.

There I was, dancing in front of thousands of people, my sweaty palms wielding gigantic pom-poms, when my eczema decided to make its first national major league soccer appearance, in front of television cameras, no less. *Really? Could I not have had even a couple of hours' peace from itching?* I wondered silently. Since I could not put my pom-poms down, I felt around the insides of the handles and found a rough surface to scratch my hand against for relief. At the same time, I shook my pom-poms vigorously, so it would look like I was excited about the action on the field.

It had frequently been said that stress could make eczema worse. I definitely felt nervous at the games and even at some of the rehearsals, but I was not going to allow eczema to interfere with the fun of being a Wowdie. I would have to learn to ignore the itching or find subtle ways to scratch my hands while performing to a capacity crowd, not an easy task.

And so it went. My eczema had become a soccer fan and was planning to attend all the games.

FIFTEEN MINUTES
OF FAME

Chapter 22

I LOVED ALL four years of my life as a professional cheerleader, which always had its perks. Many opportunities to represent the Rowdies franchise were available, from fundraisers to telethons to parades and celebrity golf tournaments. We danced at pep rallies in the malls and appeared at store grand openings. Fulfilling the requirement of five appearances per season was easy and fun. We posed for pictures constantly and our photos occasionally appeared in a local magazine or newspaper. Tampa Bay's *It's Sports! Magazine* ran a story about us that included a short bio and a photo of each cheerleader. We were treated like mini-celebrities.

I always enjoyed the free post-game concerts that the Rowdies' marketing gurus included in the price of a ticket. Screaming fans filled the stadium to hear the Charlie Daniels Band or Chuck Berry. The Wowdies dressed in special costumes for "Country Western Night" or "A Salute to the 50s." Even the dances we learned for those games matched the theme for the evening's entertainment.

We were right there in the thick of things, sometimes even going backstage to meet the band members after the shows. But along the way, I discovered that even with all the fun and excitement, I could not escape the effects of eczema.

At a game near the end of my first season as a Wowdie, we were stationed at stadium entrances as usual, to give out promotional items to fans, this time Rowdies posters. As I handed a poster to a grateful Fannie, I felt a sharp stinging pain in my hand. I looked down to see a large paper cut, the first of several. What should have been a pleasant job was soured by the annoying cuts. Of course, paper cuts were common, but more so in my case because the skin on my hands had become thinner, a side effect of my frequent use of steroid creams. I was happy when the game started, and I could stop doing what had morphed into a very uncomfortable task. Eczema always seemed to find a way to sneak into my life. If it wasn't one thing – intense itching – then it was another – dry skin from scratching.

And on a Friday morning in March 1982, during my second year on the squad, yet a new oddity appeared. Several of us gathered at Tampa Stadium to participate in the filming of a television commercial promoting the team. The producer lined us up, looked us over, and divided us into smaller groups according to height. I was in the center of a group of three. We were instructed to turn away from the camera while shaking our pom-poms, then face the camera while smiling and cheering. After practicing once or twice, the sequence was filmed and seemed to go well. The producer then pulled me from the group for a solo part.

"We'd like you to smile at the camera, shake your pom-poms from side to side, then raise them above your head," he stated.

At once nervous and excited that he had chosen me, I listened intently and did exactly what he told me to do. I then noticed that he was staring at me with a puzzled look.

"Your face is really shiny. We need to put some powder on your face for this shot," he said.

An assistant walked over to me and applied what felt like an enormous amount of powder. I tried the moves again, but the producer was still staring at me, looking perplexed.

"More powder," he stated as he motioned to the assistant again.

She dusted on even more powder. I began the steps again, but the producer raised his hand and stopped me.

"I am sorry, but your face is just too shiny and we won't be able to use you in this part."

He must have seen the disappointment on my face as he added, "You will still be in the group shot that we just did. You will still be seen in this commercial."

I stepped away from the camera as he chose another cheerleader for the solo shot. I watched as she danced the part that had been mine.

This time my unpredictable skin had prevented me from dancing a solo part in a television commercial that would be viewed by thousands of people! The Florida humidity had made my face oily and shiny, the exact opposite of my dry, eczematous hands; I wondered how my skin could be so inconsistent. When the commercial aired a few weeks later, I was grateful to see that I was indeed still in it. I received my "fifteen minutes of fame" when friends called to tell me they had seen me on television. The commercial aired for months, during the Rowdies soccer season. My disappointment in losing the solo part faded and all that remained was the memory of a fun day and unique experience.

As the eczema continued to ebb and flow, I had to tackle it as best I could, while patiently keeping the promise to myself that I would not let eczema get in the way of enjoying my time as a Rowdies cheerleader. Eventually I mastered the artful combination of pom-poms, paper cuts, and powder.

FLOWER POWER

Chapter 23

IN 1983, REDBOOK magazine published an article that would change my life, but I did not know it at the time. "Flower Power: Evening Primrose Oil," written by Dianne Hales, appeared in the July issue. The two-page report announced that studies were being conducted on the benefits of evening primrose oil to treat a variety of health problems.

My eyes focused on the paragraph that said, "Last year two British dermatologists, Drs. Steven Wright and John Burton, of the Bristol Royal Infirmary, reported that soft-gel capsules of the oil significantly improved the scaly, itchy red rash of many patients with chronic eczema." I had heard the saying, "being led down the primrose path," but I was not familiar with primrose oil. A soft-gel instead of a cream was something different. Maybe it worked from the inside out, not the other way around. I was so sick of rubbing creams on my hands and getting no results. It would be great to just take a soft-gel instead.

The article was cautionary and listed several warnings. Evening primrose oil was classified as a food supplement, not a drug. Therefore, it was not subject to testing requirements or standards of the FDA. It was sold mostly at health food stores, which were not regulated by government agencies. In addition, the article stated, "all the capsules are not necessarily created equal." Cheaper brands might have been made from the leaves of the plant and not the seeds where the good stuff, gamma-linolenic acid, was located. Primrose oil capsules made from the leaves of the plant were virtually worthless.

The author encouraged folks to buy only well-known brands, such as Efamol or Health from the Sun, both produced in England. After reading the article, I went to a local health food store and found the Efamol brand on the shelf. I bought a bottle and began taking the capsules as soon as I got home. The recommended dosage of six per day for the first twelve weeks seemed like a lot, but the capsules were small soft gels, gold in color and easy to swallow. That amount was intended for best results and to optimize the store of the ingredients in the body. I followed the directions to the letter, faithfully taking six capsules every day, either morning or evening. Some days I split the dose – three in the morning and three in the evening. I was on a mission to discover if evening primrose oil would improve my eczema.

At first I did not notice anything. I had no side effects, but my hands continued to itch from the eczema, mostly at night. Weeks went by and I still woke up in the middle of every night – scratching – until one night I didn't. I had not scratched once. My hands did not itch.

I had been told repeatedly that eczema was treatable and controllable, but incurable. Yet I was secretly hopeful, really hopeful. Another night came and went with no itching and therefore no scratching, followed by another and another. A week went by, then two weeks, and still no itching. In the past I might have had a few weeks' break and maybe even a month or two with no eczema. Perhaps the respite was just another break, a coincidence that had nothing to do with the primrose oil.

I had suffered for so long – twenty years, to be exact – and nothing had worked for any length of time. The idea that a small gel capsule could stop the itching sounded almost too good to be true. I was understandably skeptical. But deep in my gut, deep in my heart, I knew that something was different this time.

Four weeks turned into months with no recurrence. The savage, unrelenting, heinous itch of twenty years was gone – completely, totally gone. I continued to faithfully take the six capsules every day for about seven months, even longer than the indicated initial dose, just to be sure. Then I lowered the amount to only two capsules per day, as recommended for continued use. Even with the lower dose I still had no eczema. I had won the battle against the itch. I threw out most of the steroid creams, except for one that I kept as a remembrance, and in case it ever came back. But I knew that finally, I was free.

An entire year went by and I did not have one single moment of itching on my hands. The skin had returned to normal. The palms of my hands, which had been striated with thin lines from all the steroid creams, were now clear and smooth. The dryness was gone too. Evening primrose oil had cured my hand eczema.

That should have been the end of the story. But, sadly, it was only the beginning…

OFF THE PRIMROSE PATH

Chapter 24

THE NORTH AMERICAN Soccer League folded at the close of the 1984 season. Except for some minor league games, the Tampa Bay Rowdies franchise as we knew it would be no more. After four years of rehearsals and games, my cheerleading days were coming to a bittersweet end. I would miss the dancing and camaraderie with the girls, but truthfully the long hours of practice, games, and appearances were starting to take their toll. We performed one last dance at the final Rowdies soccer game in early September. Walking slowly off the field at the end of the game, I looked at the bright lights and soaked in the festive stadium atmosphere for the last time. Minutes later, I watched as a couple of the cheerleaders began to cry while they packed away their uniforms. "This has been my life," our leader said tearfully. She seemed inconsolable. Even though it had been my life also, a tiny part of me was ready to move on and try something new. I did not realize at that moment just how much I, too, was actually going to miss it.

I settled into life without the Rowdies or eczema. In place of cheerleading, my Wowdie friends and I did aerobics, went out together on weekends and relaxed by the pool in our newfound free time. By then, I had been eczema-free for over a year and had actually forgotten how uncomfortable the itching and scratching had been. Eventually I stopped taking the evening primrose oil capsules, perhaps thinking I was permanently cured and did not need them anymore, or maybe I simply tired of taking capsules every day. Either way, this casual offhanded decision would turn out to be a huge regret.

My librarian job at the SmithKline Laboratory was going well, providing a steady paycheck and good health insurance. All that changed one day when my supervisor stopped by my desk in the library.

"We may be making some changes in our operations and staffing at some point, and possibly closing the library within the next year or so. I wanted to let you know…" His voice trailed off.

"Thank you for telling me," I replied. I was a bit surprised by this turn of events, but the laboratory had new leadership, so some changes could be expected. I appreciated my supervisor's warning that the library might close and I could lose my job, but I still panicked, out of concern that there might not be other library positions available in the area. I updated my resume and threw myself into a job search.

DON'T BUG ME

Chapter 25

WEEKS WENT BY and none of the advertised jobs appealed to me. I decided to broaden my search beyond corporate library positions. Meanwhile, my work at the laboratory continued. Although I had been assigned new tasks and the job appeared stable, I still felt that the library could be closed at some point. I kept looking for other options.

I was still free of eczema and never gave it a thought. So I was surprised late one night when my left hand began to itch as I climbed into bed. Gradual and inconsistent at first, I ignored it. But a few weeks later, when the itching increased, I automatically reached for a half-used tube of steroid cream, which I dragged from the back of a drawer and rubbed on my hand. Somehow, the primrose oil cure did not even occur to me then. My thoughts were totally elsewhere. I was anxious to find a job and would deal with the eczema recurrence another time.

As 1984 came to a close, I applied for a sales rep position at a local pest control company. I was quickly granted an interview despite having no marketing experience. Perhaps it was the Rowdies cheerleader gig that I always included on my resume, thinking that it would make me appear well-rounded, outgoing, and community minded.

The interview started out well. The recruiter was a man in his forties who had some prominent role in the company. He was very pleasant and listened intently as I explained that I wanted to change careers and that I would make a good sales representative. Confidently I described myself as outgoing and driven to succeed. He seemed to believe in me. I felt excited thinking that he might actually offer me the job on the spot.

The recruiter brought out some forms to explain what a typical day with his company would be like. "You will be lining up accounts for the company. Since we live in Florida, pest control is a major business and just about everyone needs some type of exterminator service for homes and offices. Our company is very well known and getting new accounts will be easy," he stated.

"That sounds great," I responded.

He then added, "After you get the account, you will set up appointments for the pest control with our main office. Then on the day of the appointment you will go into the home or business and spray for pests. You will use different types of products for different types of insects."

What? My enthusiasm came to a screeching halt.

He continued detailing the types of sprays and treatments that would be used to eradicate various pests, including ants, bees, wasps, and roaches. *Ah yes, my friends from the dormitory – roaches.*

He rambled on, but I had stopped listening.

How could a sales representative job include the actual spraying of the buildings? I wondered.

It sounded like false advertising to me.

Boldly, I stopped him mid-sentence. "So, I would actually be doing the spraying?"

"Yes," he answered.

"I don't want to do the actual spraying of the buildings. I thought this was a sales rep job. I just want to be a sales rep."

"Well, spraying the buildings is part of it. It's part of this job," he replied.

There was silence.

After a few seconds, I conceded. "Okay, I understand that spraying is part of the job. I will think about it." I wanted to be professional and could always turn the job down later if it was offered to me.

I thought about breathing the spray. I thought about my eczema that had suddenly reappeared. I pictured it getting worse handling chemicals and inhaling the various substances. I visualized getting eczema over every inch of my body, from my toes to the top of my head. I imagined myself dying from eczema, something that has never happened to anyone, ever. I would be the first. It would be my legacy – I would die from itching and this job would be the reason.

A few seconds passed and I knew I had to tell the truth.

"Actually, I really do not want to be involved in the spraying of buildings. I am sorry, but this is not the job for me. Thank you for your time."

He looked directly at me and seemed disappointed. To my knowledge, bug spray had never been linked to eczema, but I was not willing to take the chance. I was proud that I had been true to myself and spoken up, even if it meant losing the job offer.

Back to square one.

DREAM JOB

Chapter 26

ONE SUNDAY IN February 1985, my job-hunt luck finally changed. A large ad announced that Shriners Hospital for Crippled Children would be opening in Tampa later in the year. (The word "crippled" was later dropped.) At the time there were nineteen Shriners Hospitals in the United States, plus one in Mexico and another in Canada. This new location would be a state-of-the-art facility, and like the other hospitals would provide world-class orthopedic care for children regardless of the family's ability to pay. Shriners Hospitals had a wonderful reputation, and the care of the patients was known to be exceptional. I quickly scanned the posting looking for anything that might fit my talents – nurses, operating room staff, secretaries, a dietician, a social worker. There was nothing I qualified for. And then I saw it. A hospital librarian was on the list! I had feared that there were no library jobs available in the area, and suddenly one appeared that looked like the perfect fit. I immediately sent in my resume.

Two weeks later, I received a phone call that seemed to be someone from the hospital.

A male caller asked, "Are you looking for a cheerleading job? We have an opening for a cheerleader at Shriners Hospital."

What? Is this some sort of prank?

A few people knew that I had applied for the library job at Shriners Hospital. Was one of them pretending to be from the hospital and mentioning cheerleading as some sort of joke? As usual, I had included Rowdies cheerleading on my resume. But I certainly did not expect it to be the first topic of conversation when applying for a job.

"Who is this?" I responded briskly.

At that point the caller sounded more serious, and asked if I could come to the hospital later that week to interview for the library job. Perhaps this was not a joke after all. I agreed to the interview, still not 100 percent sure that it had been someone from the hospital calling me.

As it turned out, the mystery caller was actually the Chief of Staff of the new hospital. He had a style all his own, with a decidedly great sense of humor. At the interview, he showed me the space where the library would be located. It was still a shell, with concrete floors and unpainted walls. I saw rows of empty shelves and a big circular desk that housed a pleasant office area. Several large windows lined one wall and overlooked a pond surrounded by trees. Despite the unfinished appearance, the space was bright and inviting. The medical librarian of the new hospital would have the opportunity to create a library from the ground up.

I was delighted to learn from the chief that the new job mirrored not only all of the current tasks that I loved at SmithKline, but also provided many new technical and leadership opportunities to take my skills to the next level and beyond. Besides the basic responsibilities of building a book catalog and check-out system, conducting literature searches, finding journal articles, and purchasing books for the medical staff of physicians, nurses, and researchers, the position included several other important tasks. I would also have some responsibility for coordinating continuing education programs for hospital employees, assisting patients and families with searches for medical information, managing the library budget, and promoting the library to all staff. The title of the position was actually Coordinator of Professional Educational Resources, which sounded great to me. I learned that I would be considered a department head and expected to attend various management meetings. It was all right up my alley. Best of all, if offered this job, I would become one of the founding employees of this amazing new hospital. It was an incredible opportunity. Although the chief seemed positive, he indicated that the position was not yet finalized and that he would be in touch with me.

I left the interview ecstatic. This was indeed a dream job, and I hoped and prayed it would be *my* dream job. Although for a time I had expanded my job search outside the field of library science, being a librarian was truly my passion and my first choice. I felt optimistic that the position would be approved and that I would be the lucky one to land it.

DOWN THE PRIMROSE PATH

Chapter 27

THREE WEEKS LATER I had not heard anything more about the job. Nothing. I decided to call the chief to inquire if any progress had been made toward finalizing approval of the job, and to show my continued interest in the position. He took my call and said that nothing had been decided yet, but he would let me know as soon as a decision was made. He sounded confident and I was glad that I had called.

By June it had been over three months since my interview, and understandably I was becoming concerned and anxious. *What if they don't approve the position? What if he decides to hire someone else? Wouldn't he call me if this isn't going to work out? Will I need to start looking for other jobs again?*

Fortunately, my job at the laboratory was going well, but I was still counting on my dream job coming to fruition. And on top of everything, eczema covered my hands again. Maybe it had come back to join me in resuming my job hunt, or perhaps it wanted to be noticed as I shook hands with potential employers. "Hello, I am

Claire's hand eczema and I will be working with you also. It's nice to meet you."

The increased itching on my hands reflected my angst. Once again, the steroid cream did nothing to help. My eczema laughed in its face. Twenty years of Itch. Scratch. Repeat. It was a familiar vicious circle. I had been so distracted by my on-again, off-again job search that it still did not occur to me to reach for anything other than my go-to remedy, until my cousin reminded me that taking the evening primrose oil had stopped the itching previously. I suddenly realized that I had turned to the steroid cream without even thinking about what had actually worked for me before. Although there was no explanation for this odd lapse in my memory, I wasted no time in purchasing a bottle of evening primrose oil at the drugstore. Not finding the Efamol brand right away, I settled on an unfamiliar brand, figuring it was better than nothing. I immediately downed six capsules.

After four weeks there was no improvement, so I stopped taking the primrose oil. I still had the eczema, my hands still itched, and I was puzzled. The primrose oil had worked so beautifully in the past. I was angry with myself that I had stopped taking it the first time and wondered why it did not help the second time. Instead of the rosy cure I was expecting, I headed off the primrose path and onto a different road, fraught with uncertainty and disappointment, a journey that would take years to complete.

LIVING THE DREAM

Chapter 28

I WAS SITTING at my desk in the library of the laboratory, in early July 1985, when the Chief of Staff finally called to say that the medical librarian job at Shriners Hospital had been approved and was mine if I still wanted it. I could not hide my excitement and accepted on the spot. The job started one month later, on August twelfth. Six months of waiting had paid off, and I was ecstatic to start this new chapter in my career. I had my dream job! Solving the eczema issue would have to wait until I was settled in at the hospital.

At orientation I knew I was in the right place. The department heads already on staff attended our session, giving details about their departments, number of employees, and goals for their areas. Their enthusiasm for this new venture was contagious. Most of the staff seemed to be in their late twenties to around forty, and at thirty myself, it was a perfect fit. I saw that I would make new friends there and we would work well as a team to make the new hospital successful. Everyone was upbeat and excited about what we would be able to accomplish, and I could hardly wait to begin my contribution – building the new Shriners Hospital library from scratch.

Early on, I met with the Chief of Staff, Hospital Administrator, Director of Nursing, researchers, and others to find out their needs and what they envisioned for the library. From there I was free to do whatever it took to create a vibrant state-of-the-art resource center that would serve not only the medical staff, but also the patients and their families. My top priority was to provide requested information as fast and accurately as possible, no matter how obscure it might at first appear: "I recently saw an article on scoliosis treatments. I think it was in a blue journal. Could you please find it?" I loved being a sleuth and always challenged myself to crack the case, or in that case at least locate the requested article.

In time, I performed literature searches on all kinds of topics using various databases, particularly PubMed, a free database produced by the National Center for Biotechnology Information at the United States National Library of Medicine. I had soon acquired enough books and journals to begin sharing and swapping resources with other medical librarians throughout the United States and Canada, and later with librarians as far away as Australia. Each day offered a new adventure to find whatever someone needed for patient care or a medical study. The job was extremely fulfilling and I felt I was making a difference. And eventually my humble start-up would be called one of the best orthopedic libraries in the state of Florida…or perhaps, *the* best.

A few months into the job, I was having the time of my life. I confided to a friend that I would still be working when I was ninety because I loved my job so much. Something fun and exciting was always happening – Children's and Hospitals Week, ice cream socials, barbeques on the back lawn, employee appreciation weeks, sports days, and holiday celebrations. From state governors to Thunderbird pilots, famous guests visited often. Even though my specific responsibilities did not involve direct patient care, I loved being part of the behind-the-scenes action. It was incredibly rewarding to see the children in the hallways or cafeteria and know they were receiving the very best care at no cost. The patients were having so much fun at the hospital, they were actually sad when it was time to go home.

For many years I was one of those lucky people who looked forward to Mondays so that I could go back to work. I felt appreciated and valued, but mostly I loved being part of something bigger than myself. The Shriners Hospitals for Children's mission was, and would continue to be, a noble one. I was honored to contribute to the cause.

ON THE RUN

Chapter 29

WITH MY CAREER on fast forward, eczema refused to be left behind. Six months into the new job, the itching on my hands became much worse. I thought that it might have been due to the strong antibacterial soap in the hospital restrooms, handling so much paper and copier toner, or maybe the stress of new responsibilities. Even though I loved the work, I did feel a bit nervous at times when learning the ropes and of course trying to do everything perfectly. My hands felt dry all the time. The moisturizing treatments the doctors continued to prescribe were ineffective, because the fact was that I did not actually have dry skin. My hands still itched and became dry only *after* I had scratched them. I was growing more frustrated with the medical profession not understanding my skin problem. Since the primrose oil had not cured my eczema the second time, and the traditional treatments still proved useless, I resigned myself to the fact that eczema could be a lifelong issue for me. Focusing on other things might be the only solution.

ജ ജ ജ

In Florida, I noticed that everyone seemed to run or jog. Despite the hot weather, runners were everywhere all the time, reminding me of how much I disliked it in college. Back in New York, I had tried running with my roommate. She jogged along happily while I struggled a few yards behind her.

"I hate this. How can you do this? It's so uncomfortable," I complained.

"Just a little further, just a few more minutes," came her cheerful reply.

After a few more attempts, I stopped joining her on her daily runs. At the time it just was not for me.

But, ten years later, in 1986, history repeated itself and another friend tried to talk me into running. Unfortunately, I was still terrible at it, huffing and puffing and taking long walk breaks to catch my breath. Eventually, I was able to run about a mile without stopping. Instead of being happy with this accomplishment, I still disliked running. But somehow, I kept on going, albeit half-heartedly. Between the job and the eczema, I needed a healthy outlet. And like anything else, with repetition and practice came improvement, although in my case it took a while.

In 1989 my friend introduced me to the Tampa Bay Runners Club. Once again I found camaraderie within a group, which I had not enjoyed since my days as a Rowdies cheerleader. I loved the socializing, parties, and supportive atmosphere. Even as a novice runner at that point, I quickly assimilated into this new bunch of confident, positive people. I listened to their conversations about training schedules, favorite running routes, and which brand of running shoes were the best for the price. I learned that they all participated in various local races from the 5k (3.1 miles) distance all the way up to the marathon (26.2 miles). They were totally into it. Their energy and enthusiasm made me want to be a part of the excitement and to enjoy the sport as much as they did.

I took the logical but challenging next step and entered a local 5k race, placing near the bottom of my age group. I envied the girls my age who could run a 5k in twenty-two minutes. They made it look effortless. Despite my poor performance, participating in the race had been fun. There was a party afterward with music and refreshments. Everyone was in a good mood and it was nice to be outside on a sunny, beautiful day. Joining Tampa Bay Runners and participating in local races had been great decisions, providing great exercise and a great social life, not to mention a great solution to my eczema-stress connection.

I was off and running.

PICKING UP SPEED

Chapter 30

POP! THE STARTING gun finally fired as I stood with five hundred other runners in November 1991, waiting to begin the Annual Bull Run, a local 5k race named for the University of South Florida's mascot. I was freezing. Although the temperature had dipped to an unseasonable thirty-five degrees, I had ditched my jacket, knowing I would warm up once I started running. The race was a milestone of sorts, my twentieth since taking up my new hobby. I wanted to do well and actually liked running in the colder weather.

After bolting out from the starting line, I tried to settle into a comfortable pace, but realized that I was running much faster than usual. Glancing around, I noticed that I was running with a totally different group of people and not in the back of the pack like I normally was. The runners looked fit, competitive, and serious. As I reached the first mile marker, I looked at my watch and saw that I had run one of my fastest first miles ever – an eight-minute mile. I still felt strong. With two miles to go, it was my chance to get a personal record (PR in runners' lingo). The second mile was harder, but I persevered. As I reached the two-mile marker, even though my pace had slowed a bit, my race time was faster than any previous race. I was motivated to keep pushing through the third mile. As I rounded the corner into the college stadium, where the race ended, I could see the timing clock ahead reading twenty-six minutes. I sprinted as hard as I could and finished the race in twenty-six minutes thirty seconds, my fastest time ever. I was ecstatic.

The post-race festivities got underway as runners mingled about, discussing their race tactics and the outcome, always supportive of each other. I listened and then shared my story. "I just ran my fastest race ever! I got a PR!"

"Wow, that's great! What was your time?" another runner asked.

"Twenty-six thirty!" I responded, knowing that for many of those ladies it would have been a very disappointing time, especially for the ones who finished in twenty-two minutes. But that did not matter to me. I had just run the fastest 5k of my life and felt great doing it.

I was excited when I heard the race director's voice crackle over the loudspeaker as he prepared to announce the race awards. I thought I had a chance to finally win one. Of course, I had never won an award at a race, but thought it might be a possibility because of my faster time. The race director declared, "We have trophies for first, second, and third place for both men and women in each five-year age group. When I call your name, please come forward and collect your award."

I was in the thirty-five to thirty-nine age group, which was usually quite competitive.

The announcer continued, "I will start with the youngest runners and move up the age groups," and began calling out each runner's name and time.

Everyone applauded as tiny children went up to accept their awards. Some of their race times were faster than mine. He continued reading the winners' names, handing each one a beautiful trophy. I wanted one so badly. He finally reached first and second place in my age group and I watched as the two women accepted their awards. He stopped for a minute and studied the results.

Do I have a shot at third place? I wondered.

He read the third-place name. It wasn't mine. My heart sank as I watched the winner walk to the front. She whispered something to the announcer, and then turned around and disappeared back into the crowd, without the trophy.

"Sorry folks, she is in a different age group," the announcer apologized, as he corrected the information he had been provided and looked at the results again.

"Third place is Claire Keneally with a time of twenty-six thirty."

I jumped at the sound of my name and rushed forward to accept the long-awaited trophy. It felt heavy as he placed it in my hand. Two years of struggle had paid off. I had actually placed in my age group at a race. I owned a trophy!

Running had become a very important part of my life. I might not have had control over my eczema, but running was one thing I could control and even improve. It was just what the doctor *never* ordered.

YOU GET USED TO HANGING IF YOU HANG LONG ENOUGH

Chapter 31

LIVING WITH ECZEMA for nearly three decades had taught me that there were two completely different strategies for dealing with a chronic skin condition. The first, and perhaps the most common, was to aggressively search for a cure, or at least for a level of control. It involved multiple doctor's appointments, various prescriptions and over-the-counter medications, specific cleansing products, and maybe special diets or eliminating certain foods. The method, which I aptly named the "Aggressive Strategy," also required the highest investment – money, time, and energy. The second and opposite strategy was to simply ignore it, and just hang on, without doing anything at all, hence the expression, "You get used to hanging if you hang long enough." This old saying, occasionally used by my mother, meant that if you tolerated something long enough, you could get used to most anything. I liked to call the second strategy the "Hanging Era."

After many years of following the Aggressive Strategy, repeatedly exhausting my supply of money, time, and energy, I had reached the point where I was used to living with eczema. My mother's saying comforted me and I invoked it regularly. When the eczema itched, I scratched it. I didn't talk about it or search for any more treatments. Nothing worked anyway. I had already tried so many brands of steroid creams and ointments, some stronger than others. I had visited multiple doctors and been prescribed the same things over and over. With no cure and no new treatments on the horizon, I lost hope. So I just hung on, defaulting to the second strategy, the Hanging Era, and did absolutely nothing related to eczema. It was a relief to simply pretend it was not there. And while it certainly was not gone, it was slightly better. I began to accept that Itch. Scratch. Repeat. might always be present in my life.

The first Hanging Era began in 1992 and lasted for nearly a decade as I went about my business, working at my dream job at Shriners Hospital, running, and going out with friends. The eczema, as always, had a life of its own. It waxed and waned like the moon, but I remained steadfast in my disregard.

ဢ ဢ ဢ

A year into that first Hanging Era I started dating Carl, who appeared to be a great guy. I was enjoying our time together immensely, until one evening as we relaxed on the couch, I began absentmindedly scratching my hands. After a few minutes, Carl blurted out, "If you don't stop scratching, I am going to leave."

Did he really just say that? You've got to be kidding me!

Instead of offering empathy, he threatened me with the loss of his company if I couldn't get my eczema under control. Never in my wildest dreams had I thought my eczema would be irritating to others. The itching was my problem and scratching was my solution. No one had ever commented on it. In fact, most people never noticed my scratching. I was shocked that it bothered Carl. Suddenly, he wasn't so wonderful after all. Carl and I eventually went our separate ways, but my eczema stayed. It was an even trade.

TRY, TRY AGAIN

Chapter 32

AFTER CARL'S EXIT from my life, I focused more on my running, which also kept my mind off eczema as the Hanging Era continued on. I competed in races whenever I had the chance. Each Wednesday night, I joined my friends in the running club for a five-mile run and pizza afterward. Five miles eventually turned into ten, only stopping for water breaks. I was still slow, but had developed the strength and endurance to run longer distances. Perhaps my tenacity and stamina from living with a chronic skin condition had carried over to running.

My trophy from the Bull Run was soon joined by a couple of others, reminders of all that I had achieved in the six years I had been running. I began to consider options for taking my hobby to the next level.

If I could run steadily for two hours, I should be able to do a half marathon, I reasoned. *And maybe I could do it before turning forty.*

I decided to try one in a nearby town, on a cold morning in December 1994. I finished the Brandon Half Marathon in just under two and half hours, enjoying every minute. Another half marathon followed, on the heels of the first, with an even faster time. I began to think that I could run a full marathon. Several runners from my club were preparing to run the January 1996 Walt Disney World Marathon in Orlando. I was excited to join them, with the goal of simply finishing it. Training for a full marathon required following a specific plan for four to six months prior to the race, and would give me control over a goal that was actually achievable, with the added benefit of providing a distraction from eczema. I was ready to commit.

The alarm clock jolted me awake at 5 a.m. on the first morning of my new training schedule. I jumped out of bed, threw on running clothes, and grabbed a coffee on the way to meet the running group for my longest run yet. Once there, I witnessed a boisterous party atmosphere. Despite the early hour, the runners were energetic, chatty, and frankly, quite loud. "How far are you planning to run this morning?" asked Charles, a fellow runner.

"I'm planning to run fourteen miles. I'm training for the Disney Marathon in January!" I bragged.

"Oh wow, that's great! I'll run with you. I need to run fourteen also," he replied.

We jogged a little slower than normal so I would be able to complete the new longer distance. We talked occasionally. Actually, he talked and I mostly listened. I couldn't breathe if I tried to do both. Eventually the conversation stopped and we concentrated on running.

I would never know exactly what happened, but one moment I was jogging along just fine and the next I was lying on the ground with a twisted ankle and bloody hands. In that split second my dream of completing the Disney Marathon was shattered. It turned out that my ankle was actually broken. My hands healed quickly. After all, they were used to being bloody from all the scratching. But the ankle took about three months to heal. I watched with disappointment from the sidelines as my friends ran the Disney Marathon, crossed the finish line, and received shiny gold Mickey Mouse medals engraved with the date. When my ankle healed, I cautiously began running again, but would not train for another marathon for six more years.

ಬ   ಬ   ಬ

The Hanging Era carried on. Eczema stayed in the background until 2001 when Protopic, a new ointment for treating eczema, was approved by the FDA. Steroid creams had been the standard treatment for decades, so this nonsteroidal product was lauded as a major breakthrough. Side effects were beginning to give steroids a bad rap, so Protopic really piqued the interest of both dermatologists and their eczema patients. After reading about the new treatment, I asked my primary care doctor for a prescription, not even bothering to visit a dermatologist. The ten-year Hanging Era was officially over. I began the all-too-familiar ritual of rubbing cream on my hands with new hope that the "latest and greatest" treatment would do the trick.

Four weeks later, after faithfully using the new cream every night, my eczema was no better. In fact, it seemed that the Protopic had made my skin worse. I was disappointed but not really surprised. Creams just did not work for me, even a breakthrough solution like Protopic. As with all the others, I tossed it aside and focused on a different goal – attempting to run a marathon again.

My desire to do a full marathon had never completely gone away. Like the eczema, it had remained in the background, emerging occasionally. When my running group announced that they were preparing for the 2002 Disney Marathon, I decided to join them once again. I started training for the 26.2-mile race, happy to realize that I had not lost much endurance. After completing several long runs, including an eighteen-miler, I felt stronger than ever. I enjoyed the camaraderie and could not hide my enthusiasm about my upcoming first marathon. But my enthusiasm soon turned to worry when the outside of my right knee started to feel tight. The marathon was only five weeks away.

"I need to continue to run to keep up my stamina, plus it doesn't really hurt," I confessed to a running buddy. "It's more just a weird feeling."

But two weeks later the tightness turned into pain. I stopped running completely and prayed for a miracle, but my knee felt terrible.

Could I still try to run the race? Was it possible to walk a marathon?

We drove to Orlando the day before the race to attend the runners' expo, as I hoped against hope that my knee would improve. I picked up my race packet, which included a colorful long-sleeved shirt with a Mickey Mouse adorning the front. I felt sick. Looking at the beautiful shirt, I knew that I would never be able to wear it if I did not actually run the race. My knee still hurt. On the morning of the race, yet again, I was not at the starting line. I would not be getting a shiny gold Mickey Mouse medal engraved with the date. It appeared that fighting eczema would be the only marathon I would get to do.

ON PINS AND NEEDLES

Chapter 33

NOT ONLY HAD I missed out on completing a marathon again, I had also lost, at least temporarily, my diversion from eczema – running. Without it, there was a void in my life. I tried to be calm as I waited for my knee to heal. I concentrated on work during the day and watched a lot of television at night. If eczema had taught me anything, it was that I could persevere. I knew I would run again, and just had to be patient during the healing process.

My knee eventually healed, and I resumed running in the fall of 2002. I had felt great disappointment and frustration when my second attempt at running the Disney Marathon had failed, but I was ecstatic that I could still run after my knee injury. Some runners had knee problems that forced them to stop running completely. I was grateful that I could continue enjoying the sport that, amazingly, I had grown to love. Disappointment and frustration continued, however, with the other marathon in my life – eczema. On New Year's Day 2003, I realized that I had been putting up with eczema for forty years. Living with it was indeed a marathon, but one without a finish line in sight.

For some unknown reason the eczema on my hands had been increasing in severity over the last several months. More frequent itching, especially at night, was affecting the quality of my sleep. Since the Hanging Era had officially ended, I decided to revert back to the first and more common strategy of dealing with a chronic skin condition – aggressively searching for a cure, or at least a level of control. The intensity and duration of the eczema at any given time dictated which strategy I chose to follow, making me feel like a ping pong ball in a frenzied game of table tennis. Returning to the Aggressive Strategy also required a significant reinvestment. Little did I know exactly how much money, time, and energy would ultimately be demanded.

First on my list was alternative medicine to treat my eczema, specifically acupuncture. My cousin had recommended it, as she had found some success with the procedure for treating her frequent headaches. So I searched for a qualified acupuncturist, preferably a physician who had actually studied in China and had years of experience. After calling a couple of them, I was truthfully told that acupuncture might not help eczema, but I wanted to try it anyway. Quite frankly, I was curious, and there was still the small possibility that it might work. My childhood fear of needles had subsided, I had outgrown my previous treatments, and I just wanted to go in a different direction. Eventually I settled on a physician who met all my criteria. She sounded kind on the phone and told me honestly that it might help, but there was certainly no guarantee. Since insurance did not cover acupuncture, payment was required at each visit. I made an appointment.

Her office was located in a noisy, busy part of town, but once inside I felt a quiet peace come over me. The waiting area contained testimonials and thank-you letters from grateful folks that she had helped. I felt hopeful that I was in the right place, even though none of these testimonials mentioned eczema, but rather headaches, muscular problems, and pain. Still, I was undeterred. After a few moments I was greeted by a delightful woman who immediately put me at ease.

"How long have you had the eczema?" she asked.

"Forty years," I responded.

"Have you tried acupuncture before?"

"No," I answered.

"You will need several sessions close together to see improvement and then they can be spaced further apart once the eczema is under control."

As I waited in the treatment room, my gaze fell on various charts and diagrams hanging on the off-white walls.

How long would it take to learn all of this? I wondered. It all looked so complicated.

I began to get nervous. No one had ever said that acupuncture was painful, but my thoughts quickly took a turn for the worse as I contemplated the situation.

Someone I just met is about to stick needles in my body, all over my body. What if she misses and hits an organ or something? Who would even know? What if it really hurts? Should I stick it out or jump off the table and run?

Fortunately, at that moment, the doctor returned, interrupting my anxious thoughts.

"Let's do this," I heard myself say. I watched, mesmerized, as she slowly inserted the first needle into my leg. I felt the needle slightly, but it was definitely not painful. I began to relax. She inserted more needles, several into my legs and a few into my stomach. She then placed some sort of herbal mixture on top of one of the needles on my stomach and lighted it. Glancing down I saw the needles glowing and smoking. I was not expecting that strange experience, but it was not unpleasant. Later I learned that this procedure was called moxibustion, and was commonly done alongside acupuncture. Specific herbs were burned at acupuncture points as part of the therapeutic process and tailored to each patient's needs. One of the needles that she inserted into my shin did cause some pain. I winced and the doctor explained that the shin area could be the origin of my eczema.

So my hand eczema is coming from my shin? I pondered that for a moment, but then concluded that the pain was probably just a tight muscle from running too much.

I was relieved when our session ended and the needles were removed. I had survived, felt fine, and no major organs had been struck. I appreciated receiving the full experience from a true Chinese acupuncturist. Eagerly I scheduled my next appointment and headed home. Later that night, I woke up twice with intense itching and ferociously scratched my hands.

Perhaps acupuncture is not an instant cure. I just need to be patient, I thought, still hopeful.

The next appointment was more of the same, minus my nervousness, with more needles and more burning herbs. I quickly hopped onto the table, feeling enlightened. Afterward, the doctor left to mix up some additional herbs for me, an extra remedy that I did not expect. She handed me a large bottle of pills and stated, "Take sixteen of these herbs every day."

"Wow, that's a lot of pills. If the eczema goes away, do I have to continue to take these pills every day to prevent it from coming back?" I asked.

"Yes!" she responded. "You would continue to take these every day."

That was more than I bargained for. The pills were not easy to swallow. It was a struggle to get them down and there were so many. And in the middle of the night I viciously scratched my hands again.

I went to two more appointments a week apart, dutifully lay on the treatment table and allowed a nice lady from China to stick sharp objects into my body. Each night after the treatment, like every other night, I awoke and scratched my hands like there was no tomorrow. I finally had to admit that after a total of four treatments, my skin was no better. I had spent over $500 on the sessions and it was time to stop. The acupuncture had been a good experience, after all, and I was proud of myself for being open to an alternative treatment, despite the fact that I could not anticipate the outcome or guarantee results. Even if the acupuncture had worked, it would have been difficult to keep up with so many pills and appointments. The doctor had been kind and had really tried to help me, so I called to tell her thank you, but I would not be back. I had to face the fact that acupuncture did not work for eczema – at least not mine.

DOWN THE PRIMROSE PATH...AGAIN

Chapter 34

THE FAILURE OF acupuncture to improve my skin condition left me without another clear alternative medicine option, at first. Eczema was still plaguing me. Suddenly it occurred to me that the one and only remedy that had worked in the past was evening primrose oil. Until I stopped taking it, I had been eczema-free for nearly two years. I could not get the thought out of my head that the primrose oil capsules had totally eliminated the eczema when I was in my twenties. Equally puzzling was that the primrose oil had not worked when I tried it briefly a few years later, perhaps because I had used a generic brand. I considered trying the capsules again, recalling that the Efamol brand of evening primrose oil was the one that had actually worked. So in April 2003, one month after the acupuncture fail, I located the Efamol brand of primrose oil at a local health food store and purchased two bottles. A bottle had enough soft-gel capsules for one month, if I took six a day, which was the dose that had worked the first time. I figured

I would try it for a month or two. It had taken about five or six weeks to see improvement the first time I had taken the capsules – or so I thought. I did not consult with a doctor, nor did I read the instructions on the bottle. I just followed my own instincts, based on a vague memory. I faithfully took the six capsules every day, never missing a single day.

Six weeks and a bottle and a half later, the eczema was no better. Extremely disappointed and still baffled by the lack of improvement, I concluded that it wasn't even worth taking the rest of the capsules for two more weeks to finish off the bottle.

ECZEMA CREAM: APPLY. SCRATCH. REPEAT. AND REPEAT AND REPEAT...

Chapter 35

SINCE TWO ALTERNATIVE medicine options had not worked, I decided to try traditional medicine again and found a dermatologist in the Tampa Bay area with an outstanding reputation. It took months to get an appointment with "Dr. A," but I hoped it would be worth the wait. When I called in early June 2003, the first available appointment was in November. I was astounded and excited at the same time. I thought he truly must be an incredible doctor to be so busy with patients that it took nearly six months to get in to see him. I felt extremely hopeful that he might have an answer to my problem.

At the long-awaited appointment in November, I filled out the obligatory paperwork once again – eczema, chronic, since the age of eight, mostly hand eczema. After an hour's wait, the nurse called me back to a room where I sat alone for a few minutes. Finally,

Dr. A sauntered in. He quietly said, "Hello," and began reading the paperwork I had completed, but I was eager to get the ball rolling.

"I have had eczema for forty years and I have tried every cream in the book and nothing worked, and I took evening primrose oil for two or three years and it totally got rid of the eczema, but then I stopped taking it and it came back and when I tried to take it again, it didn't work and now I can't get rid of it and it is driving me crazy and I got your name from a bunch of people and I hope you can do something," I rattled on.

He silently continued to focus on the paperwork. I felt oddly anxious and wondered what he was thinking. He glanced at my hands for a second and then said, "There is a new cream out called Protopic that you can try."

"I already tried that one and it did not work," I blurted out.

"How long did you try it?" he asked.

"A few weeks." I countered.

"You have to use it for longer than a few weeks to see results."

"It did not help at all and I used it faithfully," I stated firmly. "The eczema was no better."

"Well, try it for six months." And with that he handed me a prescription and started to leave the room.

My appointment was over and it was not even three minutes long. I was so angry that I wanted to scream. I had waited six months for the appointment with him, but worst of all he had prescribed something that I had emphatically stated did not work for me. I felt ignored and invisible. I looked at the back of his white coat as he turned the doorknob. "Wait!" I said loudly. "What is this for?" There were two prescriptions on the paper he handed me. "What is this other prescription?"

"It is for a stronger steroid cream. You can try that also." And before I could say anything else he was out of the room as the door shut behind him.

I was stunned and disillusioned. After pinning my hope on Dr. A, he had disappointed me. I even thought about complaining to his office staff that I wanted my co-payment money back, but of course, that was not my style. I sat alone in the room for five minutes, longer than my visit with him. His insistence that I should try Protopic again, and for a full six months, played over and over in my head. I began to wonder if he might be right and I just needed to use it longer to see results. My gut told me that Protopic was not going to work, no matter how long I used it. But I was running out of treatment options, both traditional and alternative.

On the way home I got the two prescriptions, and that night began the familiar ritual of rubbing cream on my hands. As usual I woke up four or five times, itching and scratching. Night after night I applied the Protopic and night after night I scratched. After two months my hands were worse than they had ever been in my entire life, and on top of the itching, they had become swollen and raw. The obedient child I once was became the obedient adult, following doctor's orders exactly as prescribed, but with unbearable results. With four months of the prescriptions left based on Dr. A's recommendation, I could not take it any longer. Finally even my inner child rebelled. I stopped using the Protopic, tossing it into my cache of other creams. By pinning all my hopes on this doctor, I had wasted eight months – six waiting for the appointment and two more trying a useless and damaging treatment. My reserves of money, time, and energy, required by the Aggressive Strategy, were running low. I again found myself out of ideas as well as dermatologists.

A week later, a solitary thought came to me in the middle of the night: the dermatologist's expertise could have been in an area other than eczema. I later learned that his excellent reputation was indeed accurate and well-deserved, perhaps just not in the treatment of eczema. I promised myself to seek out only eczema specialists in the future.

MORE PINS AND NEEDLES

Chapter 36

AFTER THE DISMAL outcome and disappointment with Dr. A, another conventional treatment opportunity came up. One day my runner friend, Brittany, casually mentioned that she would have to miss our next group run to get her weekly allergy shot. "I am allergic to all kinds of things and the allergy shots are helping," she explained. "I have been getting them for months and want to see the treatment through."

I then disclosed that I had undergone allergy patch testing years ago to see if allergies were causing my eczema. "The test was a three-day nuisance that revealed I was allergic to some obscure industrial compound that I had never heard of, let alone used. Another colossal waste of time," I stated. In my opinion, allergies were not causing my eczema.

"A lot has changed with the testing and treatment of allergies," Brittany offered. "Maybe now there would be something new that would help you. Allergy testing has come a long way and maybe you should give it another chance."

Her suggestion ran through my mind. I had recently discovered, quite by accident, that I might have an allergy that patch test hadn't identified – to latex. While washing dishes I always wore rubber latex gloves to protect my hands from the dish detergent, thinking that I was saving my skin from the harsh chemicals of the dish soap, but actually it was quite the opposite. I started to get eczema on my wrists where the rubber touched my skin. I also remembered the rubber boots that I wore as a child, and that eczema had suddenly appeared on my feet at the same time. It was a revelation! When I stopped wearing the latex gloves, the eczema on my wrists went away. I thought there was a strong possibility that if I were allergic to latex, there might be other allergies as well. So to find out, I called Brittany's doctor the following week.

"This type of allergy testing will be different from patch testing with tape," the allergy doctor explained at my first appointment in February of 2004.

"Needles containing various allergens will be placed in your forearms. If you are allergic to anything the skin becomes irritated, turns red, and possibly swells. Then we might have some answers. We check your arms every few minutes for a reaction to the allergens," he stated.

I had lived through the acupuncture so this would be a piece of cake. And I was curious about the outcome, wondering if allergy testing would finally reveal some secret answer to my eczema mystery. I was actually looking forward to getting poked with a bunch of sharp objects again, hoping for lots of irritation, redness, and swelling skin.

What is happening to me? I wondered.

Solving the eczema problem had become some sort of peculiar hobby.

At the second appointment, a nurse did the actual allergy testing. She placed a grid with various allergens on my forearms, waited a few minutes for my skin to absorb them and poked each spot with a sharp needle. It was uncomfortable but not really painful, and over quickly. I couldn't wait for red spots to appear so that I could discover what was causing my eczema. The nurse left the room and I stared at my arms. Nothing. Two minutes later she returned to check my arms. Nothing. No reaction to any of the allergens. The nurse left again. I stared at my arms again. Nothing. Still no reaction. Ten minutes later, there had been two more visits from the nurse and still nothing. If I had allergies, they were mild. Most people with severe allergies would have had a fast and strong reaction to the testing. The skin on my arms still looked normal.

Finally, I saw a few light red patches forming, very slow and barely visible reactions to some of the allergens. The doctor concluded that I did have some allergies and could start a program of allergy shots, adding that eczema did not always improve with these shots. He emphasized, "Eczema is a tricky thing. There is no guarantee. You can think about it. In the meantime, here are some samples of prescription antihistamines to try. These are stronger than over-the-counter medications, and they may have some side effects."

He gave me some literature with all kinds of allergy advice and products to buy – special air filters, vent covers, a different type of vacuum, sprays to neutralize dust mites, powders for the carpet, laundry detergent add-ins, devices to control humidity and prevent mold, and encasings to wrap the mattress, box springs and pillows. The list went on and on. Following all this new advice would have been like having a second job. It was just not going to happen. I decided to try the antihistamines, but was not about to buy all those recommended products, constantly clean my place, and wash clothes a certain way. More importantly, my gut feeling told me that I really did not have allergies because I had not reacted to the prick test quickly or severely enough. And even the doctor himself had pointed out that eczema was a tricky thing.

I took the samples of antihistamines home and laid them out on the table. I was given Clarinex, two types of Allegra, Singulair, Zyrtec, and two that I had never heard of, Palgic and Rynatan. I wondered if any of these medications would stop the itching.

This could actually be fun, I thought to myself. *Another eczema experiment – and this one doesn't involve needles!*

Of the seven different kinds, there was enough to take each medication for two days. If there were any side effects, I needed to wait a day before trying a different medication. Some would make me tired. Some might make me irritable or mean. Some might even cause bizarre behavior. Maybe that was okay. I was already pretty bizarre with all my itching and scratching. Who would even notice a difference?

I faithfully followed the directions, taking the required dose for two days and logging the side effects. The pills that helped a bit made me tired. Others did nothing to stop the onset of itching. They all seemed to have some sort of side effect – tiredness, dry mouth, even some dizziness. Quickly, I gave up on the idea that these prescription drugs were the answer to my problem. Once again, my instincts took over and I did not go back to the allergist. I had learned to trust my intuition after so many years of trying to find a solution to my problem. I did, however, throw out my latex rubber gloves.

PALMING FOR ITCHY PALMS

Chapter 37

AS I CONTINUED to run my eczema marathon, still following the Aggressive Strategy, I was determined to go the distance. With the failure of two conventional medicine treatments, Protopic and allergy testing, and two non-traditional treatments, acupuncture and the short stint with evening primrose oil, I was running out of ideas. Having reached the point of no return, I became willing to try anything, no matter how unorthodox, unproven, or downright strange.

Joe, a friend who worked with me at Shriners Hospital, knew of my struggle and empathized with me. He had heard of a new therapy for eczema – palming the calves. A quick internet search provided some information on this unusual therapy. One website stated that palming the calves could help regulate body temperature which could rejuvenate the skin. In Eastern medicine, too much heat in the body was thought to contribute to eczema. It made sense. Joe was up for the role of therapist to help me try this new treatment. The twenty-minute therapy required Joe to place the palm of his right hand onto my left calf and his left hand onto my right calf, which sounded to me like a game of Twister™. We began the unusual treatment, and chatted about work and hobbies as the time passed quickly.

The next day we tried another twenty-minute session. That time, Joe thought he felt a force or energy in my calves; perhaps the eczema was leaving my body through his palms. I, on the other hand, felt only guilt about Joe's arms getting sore from keeping them in one position for so long. And I had to admit there was no improvement in my eczema. We agreed that this treatment would be too difficult to keep up and our second session was our last.

I had appreciated Joe's empathy, even if our experiment had not solved the problem. I knew that two of my co-workers at the hospital had put up with eczema for almost as long as I had, although we rarely discussed it. I decided it was time to talk about eczema with these two friends in the hope that we could help each other. To compare notes, we began a weekly lunch meeting that quickly evolved into a support group. We shared information about treatments, new creams on the market and how tired we were from scratching all night. It made me feel less alone on my eczema journey.

I learned that Linda's eczema was different from mine and more widespread than just her hands. She had some itching, but extremely dry skin was her main complaint. Like I had, Linda visited multiple doctors and tried every therapy in the book. Kara's eczema was predominately on her hands, but with only occasional itching. She thought allergies had caused the onset of her eczema.

The talk was fun at first. We called our group the "Eczema Buddies." I looked forward to commiserating with them, although we never really solved anything. Eventually, we realized there was only so much one could say about eczema and we became tired of dwelling on it. After two months we ended our support group, promising each other that if one of us found a successful treatment we would reconvene the Eczema Buddies to share the discovery. Even though we stopped talking about eczema, our group had achieved its goal. Sharing our struggles had provided comfort to each of us.

A LITTLE HELP
FROM MY FRIENDS

Chapter 38

THE TAMPA BAY Runners Club provided a welcome respite from the reality of fighting eczema. As with all the other groups I had gravitated toward in the past, the common denominator was clear – a unified purpose, friendship, camaraderie, and encouragement that unfailingly greeted me from the moment I joined each of them. Running had become my therapy, providing a healthy diversion and a busy, vibrant social life. In spite of the disappointments with my two marathon attempts, I still had endurance for running. I knew I wanted to train for a marathon one more time.

At first, I did not tell anyone in my running club. I just ran every chance I got. My long runs gradually increased from ten miles to twelve miles, then to fourteen. I did not fall, I did not get injured, I just ran. I had developed stamina for the long haul. Eczema had taught me persistence, tempered with patience. After a sixteen-mile training run I felt ready to share my goal. As always, my trusty running group was right there for me with the perfect idea. "Don't try the Disney Marathon again – too much bad luck for you with that one. Disney is not meant to be for you," a friend warned. "The Jacksonville Marathon is coming up in December. It is usually cooler and the course is flat. A whole group of us will be going up. You can join us. I know you can do it." Her words were the extra incentive I needed.

On a cold Sunday in December 2004, I boarded a shuttle bus for the starting line of the twenty-second annual Jacksonville Marathon. To say I was nervous was an understatement. I barely slept the night before, which was really not a good thing when I was about to run twenty-six miles. But I felt more determined than I had ever been about anything in my entire life. The cold temperature was perfect for me. I was injury-free and I even had friends there supporting me. After two cups of strong coffee, I was more than ready – stoked and shaking with excitement. I stood in the starting corral soaking it all in and mentally getting ready to test the limits of my endurance – confident, yet still scared out of my wits.

I'm actually here! I have made it to the starting line without injury, I thought. *Now I just have to finish this race.*

The starting gun fired and I took off rapidly, staring down at the ground as usual to avoid tripping. Suddenly all the runners in front of me abruptly stopped. "A false start!" someone shouted.

You have got to be kidding me! I thought, as we regrouped at the starting line. *How ironic! Am I ever going to get this thing started?*

A minute later, *finally*, I was on my way.

Most marathons provided water stops every mile or two. Slower runners, like me, typically took a cup of water and walked for a moment to drink it, then resumed running. But on that day, I grabbed the cup of water and kept on going.

I cannot waste one second on anything except moving forward, I thought as I tried to down the water while continuing to run. The first few miles went by quickly. I felt good and strong, getting there, inch by inch, mile by mile. But by mile thirteen I began to tire, and I was only half done. With my confidence waning I wondered, *Is this really more than I'm capable of?* I took an ibuprofen as a cautionary measure, not wanting pain of some sort stopping me. However, it was actually my mental state that was beginning to deteriorate. I was getting worried about completing the marathon.

At mile fourteen, I noticed some walkers near me. It appeared that somehow, they were walking and running the entire thing. When they walked, I caught up to them and passed them. When they began running again, they would catch up and pass me, only to stop and walk again. We went back and forth like that for three or four miles. Then it dawned on me that they were getting a nice walk break and there I was pounding my legs on the pavement, step after step, in what had become a slow, ugly jog. I never really gained any ground on them. They were always somewhere near me, running for a minute or two and then walking for a minute or two. As they walked, they chatted. I overheard their discussions, peppered with laughter.

How could this be happening? I wondered. In the middle of a test of endurance and the human spirit, the group was having a fun time and joking around. They were actually *enjoying* the marathon while I was slowly becoming a mental case, riddled with negative thoughts and a new fear of not being able to finish the race.

It was time to join them. I knew I couldn't finish the race without support from somewhere. I hoped this group of runners would be the answer. The next time they walked, I stopped running and walked with them. They welcomed me with open arms. "This is my first marathon. I'm just hoping I can finish," I said. "I have to finish this! I have to!" I emphasized loudly.

"You will finish this," one of the women replied. "I can tell by the look of determination in your eyes that you will finish."

Her vote of confidence amazed me and I instantly felt better. The encouraging group of runners provided the mental boost I craved and the support I hoped for. They explained that they ran marathons together all the time, using the same pattern of walking for a minute or two, then running for a minute or two, repeating the walk-run pattern throughout the entire marathon. I learned that their technique, called the Galloway Method, reduced fatigue and lowered the chance of pain or injury, enabling thousands of people to complete marathons. I had never tried it before but it certainly proved to be the ideal solution to my marathon angst.

As we walked, we chatted about many things – good places to run, other marathons they had done, and upcoming races they were planning to do. In reality, *they* chatted about many things. I pretty much listened. I needed to catch my breath during the walk portions since the running pace was faster than I was used to. At mile twenty-five, I knew I would make it. With just one mile remaining, I would have crawled on my belly if I had to. The wonderful group of runners stayed with me for the final mile, a true random act of kindness, because they could have sprinted in.

As we rounded the corner to enter the high school stadium where the marathon finish was located, the runners warned me of an uneven area of sand and gravel ahead. It stretched before me, precarious on a good day, but particularly treacherous at the end of a grueling twenty-six-mile run. Crawling on my belly might actually have been a good idea at that point. The group jogged ahead of me, increasing their speed as they entered the stadium. I stayed a bit behind, cautiously taking each step, my eyes glued to the ground to avoid falling. All that was left to the finish line was a one-quarter mile loop of the track.

Then it was my turn to enter the stadium, to finish what I had started so long before. The setbacks of the past would not mean anything. At last I would feel that marathon medal around my neck. Even if it was not a Disney Marathon Mickey Mouse medal, it was still worth every second. I crossed the finish line in four hours, fifty-six minutes and forty-five seconds. I was finally a marathon runner, with a little help from my friends.

SEEING THE LIGHT

Chapter 39

SETTING THE GOAL to run a marathon and finally accomplishing it had required trial and error, endurance, and support, much like my battle with eczema. I hoped my successful Jacksonville Marathon journey would also carry over to my eczema marathon journey. Since the Hanging Era ended, I counted five unsuccessful sprints in the eczema marathon – Protopic, acupuncture, a quick round of evening primrose oil, allergy testing, and palming the calves. Despite these disappointments, I found myself continuing to aggressively search for a cure for my eczema, or at least some level of control. In addition to the money, time, and energy already invested, even more trial and error, endurance, and support would be required to reach the goal. My success at the Jacksonville Marathon gave me a renewed sense that I should not give up. If eczema was a marathon journey, so be it. I would endure.

In February 2005, two months after my marathon, a new dermatologist prescribed the standard creams, which of course did not work. He also suggested a product I had not tried before – Olux Foam. It came out like hair styling mousse when I pressed on the dispenser, and the fluffy foam did help a bit to stop the itching, but it still did not prevent the itching from starting in the first place. Then the dermatologist recommended using a "light box" to treat my eczema. Also called phototherapy, the light box was a fairly new treatment and had seen some promising results, according to the literature. I was just happy that it was something other than another cream.

On the day of my first light box treatment, I was ushered into a small room in the back of the dermatologist's office, which contained the special box. I sat alone in there for what seemed like an eternity, staring at the small box. It looked harmless enough. About the size of a toaster oven, it had fluorescent lights lined up in rows. In fact, it looked like a large makeup mirror, *but so what?*

If it helped, I was all for it.

A nurse finally entered the room. After exchanging pleasantries, she began adjusting the light box, turning knobs back and forth.

"We don't want you to get burned. We start slowly and build up," she stated. She continued to fiddle with the knobs. More time passed and there was more fiddling, more tweaking. She spoke again. "I am not sure about the timer and the amount of time for you to stay in it. The machine is touchy and we have been having some problems with it, getting it right."

I was not worried about the possibility of being burned by the machine, so I offered my opinion. "I have really bad hand eczema and the longer I am in the light box, the better! I really want to get rid of this."

I then placed my hands into the box as instructed, turning them palms up and then down, as the light shined on them. The nurse left the room. I flipped them over and over as the timer clicked on. The machine rattled and I felt a slight heat, but there was no pain. After four minutes or so, the timer stopped and the light went out. The nurse re-entered the room, looked at my hands, and dismissed me. I scheduled my next light box treatment for a few days later and left the office, hopeful that this new, different, and slightly unusual light therapy would do the trick.

BURNED OUT

Chapter 40

THAT NIGHT, AFTER returning from the light therapy appointment with the dermatologist, my hands felt very dry, abnormally dry, even for me. But amazingly they did not itch—at all. I went to bed even more hopeful about this new course of treatment. But the next morning, I got a rude awakening. Both my hands and wrists were surprisingly swollen, red, and scaly, but I went to work anyway. As the day went on, my hands got worse, to the point that it hurt to use them. I called the doctor's office, panicked and worried there might be permanent damage or scarring. My Eczema Buddies friend, Kara, took pictures. She had never tried the light therapy and was astounded at what had happened. All my co-workers stared at my burned hands in horror, and I became the topic of conversation for the day. "Did you see what happened to Claire's hands?" asked one.

"Yes, poor Claire!" commented another.

"Go back to that doctor's office and get them looked at right away!" begged another co-worker.

As I drove to the office, after getting an immediate appointment, I wondered why, if the machine had not been working properly, they had even used it. The nurse practitioner greeted me the second I walked in the door. She was calm and assured me there would be no permanent damage and no scarring. As an extra precaution, I was then sent to the Tampa General Hospital's Burn Unit for an additional evaluation. When I arrived, I realized they were expecting me, and I was escorted to a room at once. The hospital already had all my information, and required no paperwork or payment. I received much-needed preferential treatment, which may have been a result of the light therapy complication. The nurse looked at my hands and stated, "You have second-degree burns. But because of the eczema there is little we can do for you. It will resolve on its own."

She handed me a tube of some mild cream for burns and sent me on my way. As angry as I felt, there was one bright spot in the whole experience, however – my hands did not itch for several weeks. It was a welcome break for me.

Needless to say, I did not try the light box again. When my hands completely healed, the itching returned in full force. But as the old saying went, "Once burned, twice shy."

ENTRANCED? OR NOT…

Chapter 41

"HYPNOSIS. HAVE YOU ever thought of trying hypnosis?"

My nurse friend, Emily, had stopped by the library to borrow a book. As I helped her find what she needed, our conversation turned quickly to my eczema. After my burned-hands episode, my co-workers frequently asked how I was doing with my eczema. I appreciated their caring and concern for me, and that day was no exception. Emily sat down for a moment and suggested that hypnosis might help me control the itching and thus the need to scratch my hands. Eczema was often called "the itch that rashes," because the skin looked normal until one scratched it. It was only after scratching that the rash appeared. Controlling my mind through hypnosis to avoid scratching just might work.

The medical librarian in me came out, and I researched hypnosis and eczema on the internet and in the PubMed database. I found over thirty articles dealing with hypnosis and the treatment of skin conditions. Twenty or so mentioned eczema, with a few reporting positive results. Two weeks later I had an appointment with a physician, "Dr. H," who would show me how to hypnotize myself to control the itching of my hands. Once I had learned the technique, I would be able to use it on my own, without the intervention of a practitioner each time.

At my first hypnosis session, in April 2005, I was unexpectedly nervous. I thought about people clucking like chickens onstage or performing some other embarrassing task after being hypnotized as part of a show in some club or theatre. Certainly nothing like that would happen in the sterile environment of a doctor's office. Yet I felt some reluctance as I waited.

Dr. H strode confidently into the office as I sat fidgeting on the edge of my chair. "I will be teaching you to hypnotize yourself to help control the itching that you experience from eczema. Your particular case has been resistant to other treatments and has become intractable," he explained. I was relieved that he knew my case of eczema was very challenging, and it gave me hope that he would help me.

"Please sit comfortably in the chair with your arms resting on the armrests," he invited. *Got it.*

"Take a deep breath." *Okay.*

"Look up with your eyes at the same time as you close your eyes." *Done.*

I did exactly as he said, concentrating carefully on each step, and as I completed the final task, I burst out laughing. I glanced at Dr. H, who seemed mildly amused, but it was probably not the first time someone had found humor in the situation. I composed myself. "Sorry, let me try again."

Sit comfortably. Check.

Take a deep breath. Check.

Look up while closing my eyes. Check.

I waited for the magic to begin. What would the next step be to get me into the much-talked-about hypnotic state? But nothing was happening. I waited. Still nothing.

"Now, your arm will begin on its own to rise up off the armrest."

Huh? I wondered to myself.

My arm was not going to rise up off anything unless I lifted it up myself. I waited for a minute and nothing happened.

Were there not more steps to this hypnosis thing than looking up while closing my eyes?

Apparently not. I looked at the doctor. I wanted to laugh again, but held it in. He seemed undeterred.

"Let's try it again," he said patiently. I could hear a kindness in his voice. I sensed that he really wanted this to work for me. I tried again.

Take a deep breath. Check.

Look up while closing my eyes. Check.

"Now, your arm will begin to rise up."

Nothing. I was fully aware of what was going on. There was no magic there. My arm did not rise up. I stole a glance at the doctor.

"I will help your arm to rise up," he stated, and with that he gently and slowly lifted my arm up. My arm hovered just above the armrest, as he held it up. A few seconds later, he lowered it back down. I did not understand why he lifted my arm if it was supposed to lift itself, but that must have been part of the process. I was silent as he continued on.

"Try to feel like you are floating."

I concentrated for a moment. In the darkened room, with my eyes shut, I was surprised to find that I was actually able to do it. Encouraged, I blocked him out and concentrated again. I envisioned a magic carpet hovering in the air. I sat atop it, drifting slowly, no more gravity. I felt the floating sensation in my arms the most, which then increased to include my thighs, calves, and feet. I was doing it. Maybe I really *was* hypnotized, or at least partially hypnotized. I was still keenly aware of everything around me, yet I had the floating thing going on.

"Now, try to make your right hand warmer."

I focused on my right hand and tried as hard as I could to raise its temperature. I was really getting into it. *Heat...hot...hot water... hot sun...hot day.* Thinking of any imagery related to heat, I concentrated first on the palm of my hand, then my fingers, and then my hand as a whole. I did feel slight warmth covering my hand but did not particularly like the sensation. Too much heat in the body was believed by many Eastern medical practices to be the cause of eczema. Perhaps the temperature regulating technique was intended to address that issue. If I could tap into my body's temperature maybe I could regulate it.

"Now, try to make your hand cool," instructed Dr. H.

It was time to try to cool the heat of the eczema. So, there *was* a method to this after all. I concentrated once more. The cooling sensation was harder to get. Even after several attempts, I was unable to achieve it before our session ended. Dr. H asked me to practice the self-hypnosis twice a day for fifteen minutes at a time, until my next appointment two weeks later. It seemed like quite a bit of time to sit, meditate, and float, but I reasoned that I should at least give it a try.

Over the next two weeks I only attempted the self-hypnosis a handful of times. I could not bring myself to practice it twice a day, and several days I did not practice it at all. I got the floating sensation easily after a minute or two. It took longer to achieve the heat sensation and I was never really able to feel a cool sensation as instructed. Meanwhile, my hands still itched.

During my second visit, we went over the same self-hypnosis technique once more. I was told to keep practicing and to come back again if I needed more help. I realized that it was up to me to master the technique and devote the necessary time to it. This would be challenging, as I had never been one to sit for long periods of time. I enjoyed sports and activities that were fast moving, like running, instead of ones like yoga. Silent meditation had always been difficult for me. I tended to open my eyes and look around the room instead of sitting quietly. My mind would wander and I would find myself thinking about my to-do list instead of concentrating on the task at hand.

I resolved to practice the self-hypnosis once a day for a month, but like a New Year's resolution gone bad, I was unable to do so. I was too busy or in a hurry during the daylight hours, and late at night I was just plain too tired. And then of course, there was that other thing… Even when I did practice, the eczema was no better. To be fair, Dr. H had told me it would take a while, perhaps a couple of months of faithful practicing, to see results. He had also said that if my hands itched in the middle of the night, I should get up out of bed and try the self-hypnosis right then. I thought about it one night, as I awakened to my usual itching, but I simply did not feel like getting out of bed. Instead I scratched, rolled over, and went back to sleep, like a lazy dog on a hot summer day.

Several weeks into my feeble attempts at self-hypnosis, I received an invoice for two sessions of medical hypnotherapy at $400 each plus other lesser charges. I had no idea it would be that expensive or that my insurance would not cover it. After a few calls, I got confirmation that indeed my health insurance did not pay for those types of procedures, which were still somewhat experimental. I was told that I could appeal it by writing some letters here and there and perhaps a portion of it would be covered, but it was unlikely. Instead, I called Dr. H's office and pleaded my case, explaining that I did not know it would cost that much or I may not have gone back for that second visit. I confided to the kind nurse that my insurance would not pay for hypnotherapy, and even if I appealed their decision it did not look good. She took pity on my situation and promised to investigate. The next day she called to let me know that my total bill had been lowered to less than $600. I thanked her profusely and then asked her to let Dr. H know how much I appreciated his kindness, diligence, and sincere efforts to help me.

Eventually I realized that it was unlikely that I would return for more hypnosis lessons. The cost was too high, and worse yet, I did not seem to have the will to carry out the necessary steps to achieve the desired result. I did practice several more times, but when there was no improvement in my skin or my hypnosis technique, I gave it up.

I saved the hypnosis instructions with all my other eczema treatment paperwork in case I ever got a whim to attempt it again, but I knew that was probably not going to happen. Even though hypnosis had not solved my problem, I was glad to have tried an experimental technique so different from the traditional world of medicine that I was used to.

INSPIRATION +
RESILIENCE = RESULTS

Chapter 42

DESPITE MORE FAILURES with eczema treatments, I felt grateful that other areas of my life were going well.

In August 2005 I would celebrate twenty years of rewarding employment with Shriners Hospitals. I continued to feel extremely connected to the organization's mission of helping children. Seeing the happy patients benefit from outstanding care was as gratifying twenty years later as when I started. My dream job was still wonderful and fulfilling in so many ways.

I had the additional pleasure of interacting with many of the children and their families after I started a patient library. Books, magazines, brochures, and other materials were purchased, and filled the shelves on one wall of the library. Each contained up-to-date, easy-to-read information on conditions treated by the hospital. Though I certainly never gave out medical advice, I enjoyed pointing families in the right direction to find resources about their child's health.

Another opportunity came my way in July 2005 to work even more closely with some of the patients and their families. Shriners Hospital in Tampa hosted the National Junior Disability Championships for the first time. The annual two-week event was a sports competition for physically disabled youth, featuring track and field, basketball, archery, swimming, table tennis, weight-lifting, and many other sports. Young athletes came from all over the United States to participate, and many went on to compete in the Paralympics. Shriners Hospital employees were invited to help with the event. I jumped at the chance. I was given the title of Administrative Coordinator, assisting the director of the event with various tasks including athlete registration and awards distribution. The hours were long and I was exhausted at the end of each day, trying to tackle the many responsibilities, but I enjoyed every minute.

Halfway through the event, a co-worker and I took a break from our busy schedule and headed to the University of South Florida stadium where some of the track and field events were held. We both became emotional as we watched the wheelchair athletes race around the track to the sound of cheering fans. Despite the rigors of the competition, it was evident that the athletes were having an incredible time. Their positive energy was contagious and inspiring.

The entire experience really got me thinking. A chronic skin condition paled in comparison to the challenges many of these athletes faced. I was reminded that focusing on a cure for my eczema was just not that important in the whole scheme of things. The athletes I watched had risen high above their health condition to compete in a major sporting event. They let nothing hold them back. Resilience, endurance, and persistence had provided them with success. These skills were some of the same ones I had used when attempting to run a marathon and finally succeeding in spite of setbacks. They were also the skills I turned to while running my eczema marathon. The lesson of the day was not lost on me. Even with a chronic health problem, tapping into one's inner strength made it possible to live life to the fullest.

IN HOT WATER

Chapter 43

WHEN THE NATIONAL Junior Disability Championships ended in late July 2005, I resumed my normal routine at work and continued focusing on running in my free time. I still wanted to pursue the Aggressive Strategy of finding new remedies for the eczema. But at that point I had no clue what to try next, since the light box and hypnosis had failed...until a few months later when my kitchen faucet provided an answer.

One evening, while preparing to wash dishes in my kitchen sink, I turned on the hot water faucet. When I stuck my hand under the faucet to see if the water was hot enough, I felt a strange sense of relief. The water had become extremely hot, and as I put my hand under it I got an intense feeling of itching, but it was not like my normal itching; it was almost a pleasurable itching. I kept my hands under the faucet and the itching increased as my hands turned bright red. The strong itching feeling surged to a peak and then suddenly disappeared completely... Euphoria.

I pulled my hands away from the faucet and looked at them. The red faded momentarily and my hands felt normal. This random discovery rapidly became my newest remedy. I began running to the kitchen sink and throwing my hands under the steaming water any time they started to itch. The hot water worked almost every time. This procedure gave me an enormous amount of relief and a feeling of empowerment. In the middle of the night when my hands started to itch, I dragged myself out of bed and stumbled to the kitchen faucet to my special hot waterfall. After a minute or two, I found relief and crawled back into bed, my hands still dripping wet. Sometimes, they started to itch again a few minutes later. Once more, I left the comfort of my bed to let the hot water pour over my hands. I was addicted to the euphoria and the temporary respite that it provided.

I searched the internet to find I was not alone. Others had found the hot water solution but were voicing concern that this treatment was harming their skin as well as drying it out. Researching the medical literature in PubMed, I found nothing except one article about cleaning personnel in Denmark who had developed eczema from using a new lemon-scented detergent with hot water. It was believed that the hot water accelerated an irritant that was found in the detergent, and as a result, workers were encouraged to use lukewarm water instead of hot whenever possible. I was not using any detergent, simply the wonderful scalding water, so I continued with my remedy. At the age of fifty, I finally achieved a semblance of control and was no longer completely at the mercy of my itchiness. The natural properties of water provided a nice change from the chemicals in the various creams and from the controlled, medicinal world that I had been dependent on.

There was one problem, however, that I had not foreseen, but discovered a few days later on the last day of 2005. While attending a New Year's Eve party at a friend's house, smack-dab in the middle of dinner, my hands began to itch. I excused myself and headed to the bathroom for the hot water relief. I turned on the water and waited impatiently for it to heat up. Throwing my hands under the water, I quickly realized it was not hot enough. Agitated, I turned the faucet on as high as it would go and waited again – still not hot enough. I put my screaming, itchy hands under it anyway, but finally concluded it was of no use. My friend's hot water was never going to get scalding enough to stop my itching. Instead,

I defaulted to my usual solution and scratched my hands on the belt loops of my jeans until they bled a little. Bleeding hands were always a sign of temporary relief, and I had no choice but to wait for the first sight of blood. I began to think about other situations outside my home where the water might not be hot enough – work, restaurants, shopping, and more.

Would I need to become a hermit, staying at home just to have scalding water for my eczema?

Happy Eczema New Year! I thought to myself, and headed back to the party.

DESPERATION

Chapter 44

DESPITE THE OCCASIONAL inconvenience of water not being hot enough in some situations, the new remedy turned into my self-imposed treatment for the next twelve months, and I used nothing else on my hands except hot water. The kitchen faucet had become my best friend.

The scorching hot water continued to provide relief but also dried out my hands. Some nights I just felt too tired to get up and go to the faucet. Instead, I would scratch. I could even tell what time it was by my hand scratching.

First scratching, around midnight – found a bit of relief.

Second scratching, two hours later – frustration began to build.

Third scratching, another hour after that – time to get up and head to the faucet.

My patience was wearing thin, and the sleep disruption was really getting to me. Four decades of eczema were taking their toll. Since I had not had a decent night's sleep in months, I was tired all the time. The skin on my hands looked terrible and I worried about what they might look like when I was older. Would I have any skin left? The eczema was destroying my quality of life, and I was at a loss for what to do next. Depression seemed to be settling in. I feared I was losing control and no longer had the fortitude to cope with the eczema. At times I felt like screaming.

I confided my anguish to my cousin Marie, one of my two first cousins. As an only child, I had always valued my cousins' friendship and support. We spent some time together as children, but as adults we had gotten to know each other even better. Marie sympathized with my situation and mentioned that she had heard about a new alternative treatment for eczema that was making the rounds – oil of oregano. She kindly mailed me a bottle with instructions for use. It looked like an old medicine bottle, dark amber glass with a black stopper in the top. Three drops were to be placed under the tongue twice a day. The oil tasted spicy, like a hot Buffalo chicken wing, and had a strange taste, although not unpleasant. I added oil of oregano to my hot water treatment.

By late fall 2006, I worried that I was approaching my breaking point and decided to take the Aggressive Strategy – trying any remedy – to the extreme. As my mental state deteriorated, I felt I had nothing left to lose. I began to use multiple eczema treatments at the same time. Frantic, I dug out my "Eczema Box," a large plastic bin containing all of my treatments – tubes of creams and ointments, allergy pills, Cordran tape, over-the-counter lotions, and herbal remedies. I rubbed on two types of steroid cream plus one natural cream that I found at the health food store. I restarted the primrose oil capsules and continued to put the oil of oregano under my tongue. I popped Benadryl daily and visited the hot water faucet like a madwoman, consumed with treatments and obsessed with finding relief. I could barely keep track of what to do when, and despite my frenzied efforts, there was no improvement in my skin.

For several weeks I drove myself crazy with gazillions of treatments and the weird hot water thing. I was ready to throw in the towel. I needed to see a doctor – if not another dermatologist, then perhaps one to get my head examined. I had seen nearly a dozen physicians in the Tampa Bay area over the last twenty-five years.

Was there anyone left who could help me?

In desperation, I perused local listings for yet another dermatologist, finally snagging an appointment with someone new. My hands looked frightening and felt even worse, but I continued with my cache of treatments as I waited for the visit.

LAST CALL

Chapter 45

"DR. B'S" OFFICE was located on a sunny tree-lined street in Tampa. When I arrived at the appointment in mid-January 2007, there were already many cars in the parking lot. After filling out the paperwork, I waited in a crowded reception area. Loads of people appearing anxious and bored at the same time filled the space. I brought my Eczema Box, filled to capacity, making me feel empowered and in control. I was going to prove to this doctor that I was knowledgeable about eczema and had tried just about everything to rid myself of it.

When I was called to the back, I threw down the magazine I had been holding but not really reading, grabbed my box, and marched in, ready to do battle. I met briefly with a nurse until Dr. B entered the room, accompanied by a resident or medical student. I was not sure which and did not care, as long as I would get to state my case to the doctor himself. Dr. B looked at my paperwork and then at my bloody, scabbed hands. He asked, "What treatments are you using on your hands?"

He was probably thinking, "What the hell are you doing to your hands for treatments?" but was too polite to say it out loud.

I began the litany of my so-called cures. Then I snapped open my Eczema Box and showed him the contents. He gave a surprised laugh and asked if he could take a photo of it to use in his lectures to other physicians and residents. I readily agreed to the photo. A picture would be worth a thousand words and a photo of my plastic box with its vast array of creams, pills and foams would demonstrate just how frustrating eczema treatment could be and how far patients go to treat it. Dramatically, I began to take out every treatment from my four-decade fight with eczema, placing each, one by one, on an empty chair, until there was no more room. Like silent soldiers on a battlefield, my lineup of items spoke volumes without saying a word. Dr. B watched intently as I showed the contents and briefly explained how long I had used them. I felt validated by revealing this box to him, and he seemed sympathetic to my long, frustrating journey with eczema. As a result, I felt a sense of comfort in his presence. I had finally learned how to advocate for myself.

I asked if the oil of oregano could be making the eczema worse. He said no. I told him the primrose oil cured me years ago, but had not worked when I tried it briefly another time. He was skeptical that it had ever worked. I explained that four years prior, another doctor had prescribed Protopic for six months, and that it had made my eczema worse. Dr. B said three months was long enough if it did not help. He then instructed me, "Stop EVERYTHING. I am going to put you on Prednisone."

I questioned taking this medication, as I had heard bad stories about it and it seemed so extreme. Plus, I had never known of its use for eczema. But I had confidence in this doctor.

Evidently, I was a desperate case and at the end of my rope, so I consented to the Prednisone. Dr. B presented a progressive plan to me: Prednisone would put me into a remission of sorts. Then we would try various things – another type of allergy testing and perhaps the light box again. He said he would work with me and keep at it until I got some relief. This was music to my ears. I had regained trust in the medical profession with this one visit. I did not need to fight eczema alone any longer.

It felt good to stop all my rituals. A couple of Prednisone pills and I was done for the day. A week later, I welcomed the long sought-after relief. The itching was gone, my hands looked normal again and life was good. I went back a few weeks later to be weaned off the Prednisone, as it was not good to stay on it for too long due to side effects. Then, two weeks after stopping the Prednisone, the eczema returned with a vengeance. The itching was more intense than ever. Luckily, I had a follow-up appointment already scheduled with Dr. B, who reopened his doctor's bag of tricks to continue his plan. The next step would be another type of allergy testing, using a patch test, completely different from what I had endured at the allergist.

"Allergies can start at any age to pretty much anything, so it is definitely time to revisit this," he explained.

A few minutes later a nurse entered the room to start the allergy testing. She placed various allergens on my back, securing them with some kind of tape. I was not allowed to shower for three days. I left the office, once again hopeful for some answers. The tape was annoying and it was a little hard to sleep with this work-in-progress on my back, but I made it the three days with everything still intact.

Back at the doctor's office, I was so curious about what the test would reveal that I could hardly stand it. The nurse came in first and removed the tape from my skin. I tried to steal a look in the mirror and noticed a couple of red blotches. There appeared to be a reaction to something. Dr. B briskly entered the room and immediately stared at my back. He matched the red blotches to the possible irritants. What he said next made my day!

"You are allergic to Protopic."

"What? I knew it!" I shouted. "No wonder it did not work! It made my hands so much worse. I told that other dermatologist that it did not work and I was right!"

I felt angry and relieved at the same time – angry at Dr. A for prescribing Protopic for another six months after I had already tried it and told him emphatically that it did not work. He had not listened, nor did he test for a possible allergy to the product. I was also angry at my inner child for being so obedient and continuing to use Protopic for so long, even as it made my eczema worse. But mostly I felt relieved, because finally I had a solid, concrete reason why Protopic had not worked for me. Many of the recently manufactured pharmaceutical creams contained all kinds of ingredients, not just the main one that was supposed to help the condition. Dr. B explained that some may have had a base or emollient that could have caused my bad reaction. He also shared a valuable tip that I had not even considered. When a cream or lotion was placed on the skin, the effects of that product remained for six weeks. So even when I had finally stopped using the Protopic, the horrible effects continued on for several more weeks. This made it even more difficult to determine what was causing the outbreak. Dr. B waited for me to calm down from my emotional outburst after the Protopic revelation. He then went on to name a couple of other things I was allergic to, not much of anything to be concerned about.

"So, what now?" I questioned.

Dr. B was silent as he looked again at my chart.

"You have tried everything, and nothing has worked for you."

I nodded in agreement.

"Going forward, just use Vaseline petroleum jelly on your hands. Don't use regular soap. Use a mild cleanser like Cetaphil," he advised.

He paused again.

"You were trying multiple products at the same time. If you do decide to try a new treatment, only do one thing at a time. Try one thing only and see how it works. If you use many products at once, you will not know which one is working."

"Just do one thing," he repeated.

It made sense to me. I had been doing it all wrong. Not only had I overwhelmed my body with too many products, I had also worked my mind into a frenzy, looking for control. I needed to simplify my situation.

The best part of my appointment was the fact that I had a doctor who listened to me, offered suggestions, and thoroughly explained things. He did not rush out of the room like Dr. A had done. He seemed genuinely interested in helping me. He had as many items in his medical bag of tricks as I had in my Eczema Box. For the first time in a very long time, I felt confident that I had found the right physician. A good doctor-patient relationship was paramount, and Dr. B was as driven as I was to find relief for eczema. He was brilliant in his approach to my distress, and that made all the difference.

On the way home from my appointment, I stopped at the drugstore and purchased the petroleum jelly and cleanser that Dr. B had recommended. When I got home, I collected my arsenal of eczema products and hid them out of sight in the back of my bedroom closet, hoping I would not have to see them again. Later that evening, I started my new, simpler routine by showering with the cleanser and applying a small bit of petroleum jelly to my hands before I drifted off to sleep.

THE SECOND TIME AROUND

Chapter 46

I STOOD IN the brightly lit basketball gym in front of the judges, awaiting the results. I had just auditioned to be a professional cheerleader for one of the basketball teams in the NBA. At fifty-one years of age, I was fit and in the best shape of my life. I did not remember much about the actual dance steps that I did to get there. All I could think about was their decision.

Had I made the squad of professional cheerleaders? Would I get to wear a cute uniform and dance and cheer again?

One by one, the judges announced the names of the new cheerleaders. Several young girls in their early twenties next to me had made it. They beamed with delight, hugging one another. Then my name was called. I had made the squad. I would be a professional cheerleader again! I felt excited as we were ushered out of the gym to get our new uniforms and pom-poms…

…And then I woke up.

I had this dream sequence or a variation of it for years. Sometimes, I made the squad of a professional NFL football team. Other times, it was baseball, hockey, or even soccer again. I made the squad every time and was always disappointed when I awoke and realized that it was only a dream. In real life, no one wanted to see a fifty-one-year-old cheerleader.

Those recurring dreams were proof that I missed my cheerleading days, with the dancing and camaraderie, more than I realized. As much as I loved my running group and the folks in it, the cheerleading and dancing had been something so completely different. It was artistic and creative. Running was all about endurance, grit, and determination. It was definitely not an artsy endeavor. I missed my creative outlet and wondered if I should get back into dancing by taking a class or two, which would offer the added benefit of getting my mind off eczema again. I had been following Dr. B's suggestions exactly as he had instructed, using only the mild cleanser and petroleum jelly for a few weeks, and my eczema had improved. But it was not gone. I was happy with this slight improvement and looked forward to other possibilities that might be presented at my next appointment. In the meantime, I concentrated on other things. Perhaps a dance class would be the diversion I needed, but before I had a chance to research dance studios in the area, I stumbled upon a wonderful alternative.

On a cool March evening in 2007, I attended the Festival of States Illuminated Night Parade with a couple of friends. This annual event was held in downtown St. Petersburg, Florida, about a half hour's drive from Tampa. It featured high school marching bands, floats, fire trucks, and local dignitaries – all the trappings of a typical parade. I especially enjoyed hearing the high school bands and seeing the enthusiasm of the young musicians, twirlers, and dancers. I felt envious as they passed by. Performing in a marching band was for young people. Those days were over for me, I thought sadly. The twirlers lifted their batons high and the dancers shook their pom-poms as the parade commentator announced each high school's name. They were having so much fun.

Enjoy it now, kids, 'cause it will all be over in a flash, I thought cynically.

I got lost in my thoughts for a few moments, until I heard the crowd around me getting louder. I looked up to see a bright, colorful banner being carried, followed by groups of people swinging flags, twirling batons, and tossing rifles in the air. Behind them was one of the largest marching bands I had ever seen. Rows and rows of people playing clarinets, flutes, trumpets, and trombones marched in unison down the street. Drummers kept the beat. The crowd around me cheered so loudly that I could hardly hear the commentator announce their name – "The Greater St. Petersburg Area Awesome Original Second Time Arounders Marching Band." I looked closely at their faces. The band members were not in high school. These folks ranged in age from eighteen to eighty. They were talented musicians and entertainers, and as their name implied, they were awesome. The twirlers performed with lighted batons and another group spun sparkling flags. Like the musicians, they were not in high school, and immediately I sensed an opportunity that could be the answer to the longing I had felt for years. I needed to know more about the group and more importantly, how I could join it.

The Second Time Arounders Marching Band was formed in 1983 as a way for folks who had played an instrument in high school to have one more chance to play again as an adult, hence the name "Second Time Around." Eventually, a color guard and baton twirlers were brought onboard as an auxiliary to the band. A rifle team and flag team were also added to the line-up. The band and auxiliary practiced for two or three months, usually in the spring, and then performed in various parades and stand-up concerts. It was all voluntary, but promised an enormous amount of fun for all involved. The band provided an opportunity to relive one's high school days, only better. No one would ever be forced to graduate from this troupe. The Awesome Original Second Time Arounders, affectionately called the Rounders, was the largest permanent adult marching band in the world.

DROPPING THE BATON

Chapter 47

ON A HOT July evening in 2007, three months after first seeing the "Rounders" marching band in the parade, I attended an introductory meeting for the next upcoming season of the band. Over one hundred people of all ages crowded into the cafeteria of Northeast High School in St. Petersburg, Florida, to learn about the band and how to participate. They were mostly local folks from St. Petersburg or Tampa, but a few came from as far away as south Florida and Georgia. I learned that the band was open to anyone who had marched in a high school or college band and wanted to do it a second time. If one did not play an instrument, there were several other groups to join. The band had a place for anyone who wanted to take part, be it twirling a baton, spinning a flag, or carrying a banner that announced the group's name. I decided to join the twirlers because I had the experience from high school. Some of the groups had a few minimum requirements and held a "soft audition" to make sure members were comfortable with these requirements. Even though it had been over thirty years since I twirled a baton, I was sure I could still do it.

I soon discovered that the upcoming year held something extra special for the band. The Rounders had been invited to participate in the Macy's Thanksgiving Day Parade in New York City in November 2008. The band's typical three-month season would stretch into more than a year as the group prepared for the performance of a lifetime. The band would march down Broadway and through Times Square in front of millions of people and hundreds of television cameras. The parade was always televised all over the United States and watching it was a Thanksgiving morning tradition for many Americans, including me. Instead of sitting in front of the television though, I would be participating. It was an incredible and exciting opportunity. Life was coming full circle. I would get to do it all again – marching in a parade, twirling a baton like I had done in high school, and performing in front of thousands, like I had done as a Rowdies cheerleader. I couldn't wait to get started.

One week after the introductory meeting, I attended my first twirler practice with the Rounders band. I brought my old baton from my high school twirling days to the first practice, but quickly realized it was very outdated and too short. I made a note to self that I definitely needed to purchase a new baton. The practice began after the leaders introduced themselves and launched into the routine that we would learn. I was stunned. I had never seen those moves before. I had no idea what they were doing. The main leader, Ashley, was phenomenal. She threw her baton high into the air, spun around, and without looking, snatched it as it fell out of the sky. I did not know how to do that. In my high school we never learned to throw the baton into the air and catch it. We just twirled it and marched forward.

Ashley demonstrated some other steps and called out names for moves I had never heard of – boxcar, thumb toss, two-hand spin. I was in trouble. This was not my high school twirling group. These folks were semi-professionals and this stuff was second-nature to them. I stood in the back of the room, trying to catch on. When we had to do the steps without our leader demonstrating them, I copied the girl next to me. Not only was I unable to perform the twirling moves, I could not remember what move came next. It was my first Wowdies rehearsal all over again.

Even though I could not master a single thing they were showing us, I still felt I could learn if I just had the time. I would need a little tutoring in advanced baton twirling. I knew I had overcome challenges in the past – learning the dances as a Rowdies cheerleader when it had been so difficult at first, and finally completing a marathon despite setbacks. I did not need to be perfect just yet, but I wanted to be a part of this group so badly that I had to try to learn the routine. But then there was this other thing, a little annoying problem that was always there – my eczema. It actually hurt to twirl the baton. Although I had stopped using the steroid creams on the advice of Dr. B, my hands were still dry from having used the strong creams for so long. My skin was cracking at each spin of the baton. Even if I could master the fancy moves, I wondered how I would be able to march in a long parade, twirling the baton over and over. My heart was in it – my skin not so much. I feared a rebellion from the wrist down.

I did not want to give up yet, so one week later I found myself at twirling practice a second time. I struggled once more, and it seemed even worse than the first time. More new techniques were being added and I was just not getting it. My hands were even sorer than the first week. Things were looking pretty grim until I overheard a twirler talking about the band's dance and drill team, which was practicing in another part of the high school. My ears perked up. There was a dance team! I thought about my high school Shakerette days and my Rowdies cheerleading days. Maybe I was in the wrong group. I felt like I belonged with the dancers.

At the end of practice, I approached Ashley and told her of my frustration and the fact that I lacked some of the necessary twirling skills. She was very understanding and went on to say that baton twirling in the southern United States was completely different. The northern type of twirling I had learned in New York was military style, with lots of marching and formations. The southern twirlers used a more stylized type of twirling, something I had never learned. Ashley mentioned that the dance and drill team was still open and accepting new members. I was elated to be able to join them the following week! I felt relieved and looked forward to my first practice with the Rounderettes of the Greater St. Petersburg Awesome Original Second Time Arounders Marching Band.

One week later, I stood in the Northeast High School cafeteria practicing a kick-line with a group of twenty-five dancers. My soft audition had gone well and I was welcomed into the group with open arms. This was home! The Rounderettes performed a jazzy type of dance using sparkly blue pom-poms, very similar to the type of dance I had done in high school and as a Rowdies cheer-leader. Like the band, the dance line was composed of ladies of various ages – eighteen through the late sixties. It was not exactly cheering again, but in one way, it was better. I would not age out of the Rounderettes for a long time. On top of that, I would have the opportunity to march and perform in the Macy's Thanksgiving Day Parade, as well as local parades and events in Florida. Once again, I would have a cute uniform and pom-poms, and get to dance in the spotlight. From that day forward, whenever I awoke from a cheerleading dream, I was no longer disappointed. I was a Rounderette and that was the coolest thing ever!

FIFTEEN MORE
MINUTES OF FAME

Chapter 48

THE NEXT YEAR sped by, with dozens of dance practices and prepa-rations for the Macy's parade. There were uniform fittings, dress rehearsals, and arrangements to make for the trip to New York. I enjoyed the camaraderie with the ladies in my dance group, and these new friendships added to the fun. Get-togethers, parties, and various other social events became commonplace. I was so busy and content that any thoughts of eczema faded to the background.

I knew I was supposed to go back to Dr. B and see what else he had planned for me in his bag of tricks. He had promised he would work with me and keep at it until I found relief. I understood that he had more ideas – perhaps the light box again, different new creams, and other suggestions that I could not remember. But I was tired of trying new treatments only to watch them fail. I was tired of doc-tor's appointments and tired of focusing on my hands. Sometimes I felt guilty that I was constantly trying to rid myself of an annoying ailment. After all, so many people were in truly bad health, fighting life-threatening illness, and there I was, still complaining about itching, a seemingly minor problem. And I had to admit that my hands were somewhat better since I had stopped all the treatments. The marching band and Rounderettes kept me focused, and distracted from my itchy hands, so I cancelled my next appointment with Dr. B. I was officially back in the Hanging Era.

ও   ও   ও

On November 27, 2008, I marched and danced down Broadway in New York City in the Eighty-second Annual Macy's Thanksgiving Day Parade, as part of the Greater St. Petersburg Area Awesome Original Second Time Arounders Marching Band. There were over 500 of us – 300 musicians, 110 auxiliary members (including my Rounderettes dance group), 102 letter and banner carriers, an honor guard, and flag pageantry performers.

Three chartered planes had delivered us to New York City to march the two-and-a-half-mile parade route. After several fun days of activities, including the Radio City Music Hall Christmas Spectacular, a tour of Top of the Rock, and a dinner cruise around the Statue of Liberty, it was parade time! We awoke before 2 a.m. on Thanksgiving morning to rehearse our Herald Square segment, and then enjoyed a nice breakfast at Planet Hollywood before lining up at our assigned starting place on the Upper West Side. I got goosebumps when the loudspeaker finally announced, "Second Time Arounders, welcome to the Macy's Thanksgiving Day Parade!" as we stepped off to begin our march down Broadway.

Huge, deep crowds lined the streets, and the cheering was the loudest I had ever heard. I tried to take in every exhilarating moment. Al Roker announced our arrival at Macy's Herald Square, and our band delivered an impressive televised performance. Following the parade, we were even treated to a Thanksgiving dinner at our hotel. It was all a whirlwind experience I would never forget. Two days later I flew back to Florida, exhausted, but with memories that would last a lifetime. My recurring dream actually came true in a way that I had never imagined.

IN COLD WATER

Chapter 49

WITH THE EXCITEMENT of the Macy's parade behind me, life calmed down a bit. Our long marching band season ended in December, and as a result my dance practices also ended. Without the extra diversion of these practices, I became more aware of my eczema. I tried to ignore the itching and focus on other things. I planned a trip back to New York – not New York City this time, but to my hometown of Gloversville, in upstate New York. So in late summer 2009, I left Florida and its scorching summer heat for a two-week vacation to visit family. I enjoyed the cooler weather and the slower pace of my small hometown.

On August 20, I met my cousin Sheila and her husband Greg at the Blessed Kateri Shrine in Fonda, a short drive from Gloversville. My cousin suggested it as a way for us to get together during my visit.

I had never been to this local landmark, which was a shrine to Kateri Tekakwitha, a Mohawk Indian woman born in 1656 in Auriesville, another nearby town. As a young girl Kateri contracted smallpox, and as a result developed vision problems, as well as some sort of scarring on her skin. At age twenty, Kateri converted to Catholicism and was then shunned by her Native

American community. She would later be canonized as a Roman Catholic Saint for her great faith, with many good deeds and miracles attributed to her. When Kateri died in 1680 at twenty-four, it was said that her scarred face became clear and smooth.

The grounds of the shrine looked beautiful as we walked a circular path near the Stations of the Cross and statues of various saints. It was quiet and peaceful and we realized that we were the only visitors on this end-of-summer day. We headed up the hill toward the remnants of the old Mohawk Indian village where Kateri lived most of her life. Nearby we found a narrow walkway with a steep descent, which led to the spring where Kateri was baptized. After a careful walk down the slope, we came upon a tiny structure open in the front that had been built to contain the water coming up from the spring. Many folks claimed various cures after visiting this site and praying to Blessed Kateri.

Sheila urged me to put my hands into the spring and pray for help with my own skin condition. As a lifelong Catholic I was no stranger to prayer, but so far nothing had worked to ease the misery of eczema. I was skeptical that placing my hands into the cold, murky water would suddenly bring about a cure. But since I was right there, directly in front of the spring, I decided to follow my cousin's suggestion.

Pushing my cynicism aside, I sat down on the narrow ledge and lowered my hands into the chilly water. I mouthed a silent prayer to Kateri, hoping for a miracle, but the greater part of me was still unconvinced. I moved my hands around in the spring and lingered in the coolness of the water as a sense of peace and calm came over me. Perhaps this had not been a crazy idea after all. Like me, Kateri had dealt with skin problems and certainly could have related to my frustration. As I lifted my hands out of the spring, I felt a small flicker of hope. I had left no stone unturned in my quest for freedom from eczema.

Later that evening, my hands itched like they always did – Itch. Scratch. Repeat. I had not received the miracle I had hoped for, but perhaps I had been given serenity to accept my situation. It was certainly possible to have a happy, fulfilling life despite the discomfort and aggravation of eczema. The Kateri spring water had given me the gift of tranquility.

Back in Florida after my trip, I felt refreshed and renewed. Life was good. My job at Shriners Hospital seemed to be going well, although that was about to change. My running club was still fun, and I was looking forward to the start of the next season of the marching band in a couple of months. In the meantime, I decided to tackle some home improvement projects. While cleaning out a cupboard and discarding unused items, I came across a half-full bottle of Efamol evening primrose oil and thought about tossing it, but for some reason stopped short. Since the oil had not helped my eczema when I last tried it briefly, two years prior, I wondered why I had saved the bottle. But a moment later an even more powerful memory entered my mind. Efamol evening primrose oil had cured my eczema in my twenties. Suddenly I felt compelled to begin taking it once more. So on September 28, 2009, forty days after my New York trip, I downed the required dose of six (500 mg) soft-gel capsules. I noted the date on my calendar and then went online to purchase two additional bottles from Efamol.

One month later my hands were no better. I decided to continue the capsules for one more month, faithfully taking six each day. At the end of the second month, there was still no improvement. I checked the calendar again and verified that it had truly been a full two months since beginning the primrose oil regimen. I was still waking up at night scratching and losing sleep because of eczema. Evening primrose oil did not work anymore. There was no sense in keeping it. I held the remaining half-bottle of capsules over the trash can. As I tossed the bottle in, something occurred to me. Puzzled, I stared down at the container lying on the bottom of the can.

How is it that primrose oil worked so incredibly well for me that one time? I wondered.

There were still quite a few capsules left and I did not want to waste them.

It would not hurt to finish off the remaining gel caps, I reasoned. My intuition seemed to be pushing me to take the rest of the capsules. I pulled the bottle out of the trash, opened it, and took the daily dose, vowing to finish all the remaining primrose oil.

It was the best decision I ever made.

A NEW AWAKENING

Chapter 50

TWO WEEKS LATER, on the morning of December 7, 2009, I awoke with the immediate sense that something was very different. I had slept through the night without scratching my hands. Surprisingly, they did not itch, and instinctively I knew that the primrose oil was working again.

My hands did not itch that day, nor did they itch the next night. One week went by and then another. Sleeping through the night without itching became routine. My eczema marathon was over. I had finally crossed the finish line! I did not receive a medal for my efforts. I got something far better, far more valuable – clear, normal skin. Just like preparing to run the marathon, persistence had paid off.

Back in January 2007, Dr. B had adamantly advised me to stop taking everything for a couple of months, and whenever I felt ready to restart my Aggressive Strategy of trying treatments again, to test only one at a time. I had taken his sage advice to heart and entered another Hanging Era where I stopped taking everything and essentially ignored the eczema, this time for two and a half years. And in September 2009, when I felt ready to try a treatment again, I started by testing only one at a time.

I wondered if I might have had some divine help to end that last Hanging Era and try the primrose oil again. After all, I had visited the Shrine of Saint Kateri Tekakwitha exactly forty days before I started the primrose oil. And when I went to discard it, something had stopped me. Perhaps it was *someone*. I would like to think that Saint Kateri had something to do with my eventual "cure." Either way, I would no longer need to go to the dermatologist or get prescriptions for creams that did not work. My eczema had been healed from within. After more than forty years of suffering, my hands were finally released from the shackles of eczema.

WHY?

Chapter 51

SINCE SUCCESSFULLY ELIMINATING my eczema, I have asked myself many times why the primrose oil worked so well in my twenties and the final time, and not all the other times in between. Three things were different.

First, I had bought high quality primrose oil – Efamol. It happened to be the same brand I had used in my twenties when I was eczema-free for several years. More research has been conducted using Efamol evening primrose oil than with any other brand of primrose oil. Efamol used a gentle extraction method that removed the oil from the seeds while preserving the essential nutrients. Cheaper brands typically did not use this method and were not as effective in treating eczema.

Second, I had completely stopped all steroid cream prior to starting the primrose oil regimen. In fact, I was using no cream of any kind on my hands. Many articles written on primrose oil and eczema recommended that no steroid creams be used while trying out the primrose oil.

Third, and possibly most important, I had faithfully taken the six soft-gel capsules every day for nearly twelve weeks. In previous, unsuccessful tries I had always impatiently stopped taking the capsules after five or six frustrating weeks of no improvement. When taking the primrose oil in my twenties, I thought I had seen improvement after just a few short weeks. Possibly, at that younger age it *did* only take five or six weeks to see improvement. Perhaps, at an older age, the primrose oil needed more time to take effect. The final time, I had taken it long enough to allow it to finally work its magic.

At the time, the directions on the bottle stated:

- SUGGESTED DAILY INTAKE: 2 capsules [500 mg] per day with food or drink.
- TAKING THIS PRODUCT FOR THE FIRST TIME: 6 capsules [500 mg] per day with food or drink for an initial 12 weeks. This higher initial daily intake is recommended to help optimize the body's store of important nutrients.

I promised myself that I would faithfully continue to take the primrose oil capsules each day to prevent the eczema from coming back. I did not want to take any chances, so I ordered several more bottles and took six capsules per day for nearly a year, longer than I probably needed to. I still had no side effects and of course, no eczema. I eventually lowered my dose to three or four capsules per day, then to two per day, as directed on the bottle. The eczema did not come back. I was truly free.

A TIME TO SHARE

Chapter 52

BUT THAT JOYFUL day in December 2009, when I awoke ecze-ma-free, also held an unwelcome surprise. Later that same day, Shriners Hospital in Tampa laid off several employees and reduced the hours of a few more. I was spared from the layoff, but my weekly hours were cut from forty to twenty-four. After twenty-five years as a full-time employee, I became part-time. Despite the reduction in hours, I was grateful to still have my job in the library.

Luckily, my shorter work week did not last long. In March 2010, I was asked to work forty hours again. I helped out in other areas as needed, in addition to running the library. Some of my new duties involved data entry, and it was wonderful to be able to type and not worry about itchy, cracked, bloody fingers! Three months had flown by and I had not experienced even a single moment of itching on my hands.

I relished the freedom from eczema and wanted to share my success story with friends. The two Eczema Buddies from my eczema support group at work were among the first to find out. Our little group had not formally met in nearly six years, but we had promised all along to let each other know whenever something finally worked. I displayed my smooth, itch-free hands and showed them the bottle of Efamol evening primrose oil that had relieved the itching, encouraging both of them to try it. Even though they saw my promising results, they were reluctant at first. Finally, Linda relented and ordered several bottles. She tried it for five months but saw no improvement. Disheartened, she quit taking it. I was very disappointed that it did not work for her. Kara, my other Eczema Buddy, was still experimenting with other treatments so it was unclear if primrose oil would help her.

I also shared my primrose oil success with a runner friend who had suffered with terrible eczema over a third of her body, on her legs, trunk, arms, hands, face, and even in her ears. She began taking evening primrose oil at my suggestion and it worked beautifully for her, nearly eliminating her eczema. She was thrilled with the results and sent me a grateful text message:

"I was so miserable with eczema, I couldn't sleep. I was so tired during the day I couldn't function. I tried all the topical salves and all the other concoctions, but nothing helped. When you told me about evening primrose it was a blessing! I started taking the evening primrose. I increased the dosage until I found the dosage that helped me. Now I'm taking one capsule 1300 mg in the morning and one in the evening. I still occasionally have a flare up. When this happens, I increase the dosage…I wish my doctor had shared the possibility of primrose oil helping me!"

I was so happy to hear that she had found relief from her eczema, it motivated me even more to share my solution with others. I wanted to use my voice for good.

WRITE ON…OR NOT

Chapter 53

I HAD COLLECTED a lot of data about eczema, receipts from dozens of doctor visits, a huge box of creams and lotions, medical literature, and vast notes on treatments – enough to fill a book. So in early January 2011, when Shriners Hospital again reduced my hours, I decided to do just that – write a book about my life with eczema. I knew that my solution, primrose oil, did not help everyone, but even if it helped only a small percentage of folks it would still be worth it to tell my success story. A book describing nothing but dermatology appointments and endless lists of possible treatments sounded boring to read, or write for that matter, and I certainly was not qualified to write a medical reference book. I would leave that up to the doctors and researchers. But I was definitely capable of telling my own story. I settled on writing a memoir in hopes readers could relate to my journey, and perhaps be inspired by it. At the very least, others troubled by eczema might find it to be an interesting read.

During my long career with Shriners Hospital, I had some success writing articles and having them published in different library journals. I also wrote a short story about my participation in a triathlon, and was excited when it was accepted for publication in a 2008 issue of Angels on Earth, a Guideposts magazine. I even won third place in a Haiku poetry contest sponsored by the local newspaper. Despite this tiny bit of beginner's luck in the publishing world, I quickly realized that writing a memoir was a major undertaking and not all that easy. Even though I had a pretty good memory and all that data on eczema, it was another thing altogether to organize it into a readable and thought-provoking book. I found myself writing a chapter or two on my days off throughout most of January and February 2011, but my enthusiasm quickly waned. I was surprised at how much more involved writing a book was. I had the start of a manuscript, but not much else.

Ironically, I had endurance for other things. I had persevered with running and was finally able to finish a marathon despite initial failure. And I certainly had not given up while fighting eczema all those years, but this was different. Ten months later, in January 2012, when I was again assigned to work forty hours, all my writing completely stopped. I used my job as an excuse not to write. In the evenings I was tired from work and had no desire to sit at the computer. On the weekends, I wanted to enjoy my days off – socializing with friends, running races with my club, or dancing with the Second Time Arounders Marching Band. The book would have to wait, or perhaps more truthfully, I would never finish it.

I also questioned my own vulnerability. Was I brave enough to share personal, intimate details of my life with readers? As a quiet person, I usually kept my personal life private. Revealing my struggles with eczema publicly would require a courage and openness that I was not sure I had. I would need to put aside my self-doubt and silence my inner critic to speak my truth. At the same time, I wanted to advocate for others suffering from eczema. I knew my story and solution might help them, but fear was getting in the way. Procrastination set in. For the next six months, I did not write a single word as I grappled with doubt and apprehension. Fortunately, I continued to take the primrose oil and my skin remained itch-free and clear, but sharing my eczema victory fell by the wayside.

STRESS. STRESS. STRESS.

Chapter 54

IN EARLY AUGUST 2012, Shriners Hospital for Children did another layoff. This one was much larger and affected nearly every department. Once again, I was spared, but given many new duties. The next few months were extremely stressful, but I was thankful to still have a job. Businesses frequently resorted to layoffs, so it was not surprising that the hospital might choose to do the same. But in an organization with a smaller number of employees, the layoffs really hit home. Everyone knew nearly everyone else, and it was jarring when folks were suddenly gone. I did the best I could with the new tasks, trying, and probably failing, to keep a cheerful attitude and accomplish everything in a timely fashion. Despite the added stress, the eczema did not return. I was happy the evening primrose oil was still performing its magic.

A few months later when my hours were again reduced, I forced myself to start writing once more. Not long after, I was *again* asked to work forty hours. Fluctuations in my scheduled hours continued to occur for the duration of my employment at the hospital. Like before, I wrote bits and pieces when my work hours were reduced and wrote nothing when my hours were increased. I grew frustrated not only with the frequent changes in my work hours, but also with my lack of consistency with writing.

ဢ ဢ ဢ

In September 2015, a friend mentioned that one of her favorite magazines, *Spirituality & Health,* asked readers to share their "miracle cures." She suggested that I write a letter to them describing my miracle cure of evening primrose oil for treating eczema. I was not familiar with the magazine, so I searched the local bookstore for a current copy. The well-written articles appeared interesting and covered a variety of topics. I knew at that moment sharing my story in this magazine was an opportunity I could not pass up. Of course, I did not know if they would actually accept a submission from me, since I was not a medical professional, but I just had to try. Later that same day, I composed a three-hundred-word letter describing my miracle cure of evening primrose oil for treating eczema, and sent it in. I worded it carefully, including a disclaimer that evening primrose oil did not work for everyone. I went a step further and mentioned that I was writing a book called "Itch. Scratch. Repeat." about my life with eczema. It was the first time I had called myself out as a writer of a memoir. Stating that publicly was a gutsy move for me, but I hoped it might be the push I needed to finish what I had started; that is, *if* the magazine actually published my submission.

Three months later, I was thrilled when my letter appeared in the January-February 2016 issue of *Spirituality & Health* magazine, in the column "*Talk to Us*"! The moment I saw my name in print I felt validated and empowered. Indeed, my voice had been recognized. I knew I needed to finish writing the book, especially after boldly announcing it in a popular magazine. I had even revealed the title. There was no turning back. Except for one little problem–my heart still was not in it. Even though my hours had been reduced again, I did not feel like writing. By that time, I had started taking ballet classes several times a week and as it turned out, I loved it. I was not about to skip class to write. Even sitting in front of the TV was more appealing than staring at my computer struggling to put words to paper.

So days turned into weeks, weeks turned into months, and still no work on the book. The unfinished task poked at me, disturbing my peace of mind. It was always there, like an itch I couldn't scratch. I even felt guilty every time I saw a television commercial advertising a pharmaceutical medication for eczema. My natural herbal cure of primrose oil was never going to be in a television commercial, and if doctors did not mention it, most people would never try it. I needed to get the word out, but procrastination had taken over.

Something drastic would need to happen if I were ever going to complete the book.

NO WORDS

Chapter 55

IN EARLY AUGUST 2017 I was given another new project at Shriners Hospital which took a couple of weeks to complete. On a sweltering, late August morning, I finished it, dropped it off and upon returning to the library, noticed that I had a voicemail. My supervisor asked to see me in her office. I grabbed a notepad and hurried up to the second floor. When I arrived, she asked me to close the door and sit down. With a shaky voice she stated, "The hospital is over budget for the year and we are eliminating your position. You have done nothing wrong. It's just that we are over budget for the year."

Twenty minutes later I found myself standing at the back of my car piling my personal belongings into the trunk. My job of thirty-two years had come to a screeching halt.

After the initial shock subsided, I had a mixed, perhaps unusual, reaction to my layoff. In addition to a feeling of loss, I felt a strange sense of relief coursing through my body. Working at the hospital had been my dream job and I had loved it, even to the point of thinking I would never retire. I had devoted nearly my entire career to their wonderful, incredible mission that had helped so many children. But the time had come to move on.

With my position eliminated the library might possibly be closed – the library I had founded and built with my own hands. As a good friend put it, "Our hands are extensions of our heart." I had created that library with my hands – my eczema-ridden hands – and my heart. Even though much was online by then, the beauty and value of the print versions could not be discounted. I could only hope they would make good decisions regarding these resources, but I had no words. My voice no longer mattered.

Deep down I recognized that a layoff was simply a business decision on the part of the organization and I couldn't take it personally. As I exited the parking lot, my future uncertain, I wished that my dream job had ended on a more positive note. But I knew that with the passing of time, the sting of the layoff would fade and the happy memories of my all-time favorite job would remain. At that moment, however, I needed to find a silver lining and with that thought, I pressed my foot on the accelerator and drove towards home.

STORMY DAYS

Chapter 56

AS I DROVE, I thought of all the things that would be changing with my job loss. I was given only one month of health insurance and as luck would have it, one of the shorter months with only thirty days. I needed to find new insurance quickly. I had previously scheduled my yearly physical, routine dental visit, and annual eye exam for later in the year. I decided to try to reschedule each of these appointments to take place within the next thirty days, so that I could take advantage of my current health insurance. Arriving home, I made phone call after phone call explaining my situation and loss of insurance. Every single doctor's office was extremely helpful and somehow, I was able to move up every appointment. Happily, I did not need to see a dermatologist. I felt secure that those days were over and grateful that my eczema was truly gone.

There was also another issue. Months before my layoff, I had planned a trip to Santa Fe, New Mexico with a friend, who ironically had also been laid off from Shriners at another time. Our eight-day trip was scheduled for September 16, just over two weeks away. Airfare had been paid, a rental car booked, and an Airbnb reserved. I did not want to cancel the trip, but I had a lot to accomplish before boarding the plane for the 1700-mile flight to New Mexico.

And there was one more thing. Irma, a Category 5 hurricane, the strongest storm ever to form in the Atlantic, was projected to hit Tampa sometime during the first week of September, just a few days away. Many preparations were needed before a hurricane arrived, but a storm of that strength and size was particularly alarming and would require even more provisions. People were panicked, and it was evident everywhere. Processing my layoff and making a plan for the future would have to be put on the back burner as the chaos of an approaching hurricane ensued.

Later that evening, as I sat wearily on my couch, a puzzling thought entered my mind. My layoff had occurred on August 29, the anniversary of my father's death. My beloved mother had also passed away on the twenty-ninth. She had died in April a few years earlier, and though it was not the same month, there was that twenty-nine again. Further adding to the mystery was my recollection of an article I had saved out of a nursing journal. A Director of Nursing at a Florida hospital wrote about her husband who had a near-death experience while undergoing heart surgery. He had died, "visited Heaven," and was allowed to come back because he had a mission yet to complete on earth. He was also told the date and time that he would ultimately return to heaven. That date was August 29. I saved the article because it was uplifting, but mostly because the date was the same day as my father's death. It was an eerie, odd coincidence.

So instead of preparing to secure my home before the giant hurricane hit, I found myself logging onto the computer to search the meaning of the number twenty-nine. Perhaps the change in barometric pressure before the storm had somehow affected my good judgement. The hurricane would have to wait. Three major life-changing events had happened to me on the twenty-ninth, with two of them on August 29. Two deaths and the death of my long-term job all occurred on that date. Adding in the strange coincidence of the article I had saved, I knew I was on to something.

As a practicing Catholic, I had never explored numerology, astrology, or the like. Even if it was not frowned upon by my religion, I had no interest in it. But curiosity was getting the best of me. So continuing my obsession and ignoring the approaching behemoth storm, I typed "meaning of number 29" into the search box, fully expecting a numerology website to pop up. Instead, an excerpt appeared from "The Biblical Meaning of Numbers," a book written by Dr. Stephen E. Jones.

I scrolled down to number twenty-nine and there it was in big, capital letters: **DEPARTURE.**

A chill ran up my spine. Seeing this word come up on my computer screen was one of the most shocking yet comforting moments of my life. It appeared that this unscheduled "departure" from my job was meant to be. It was, without a doubt, the time to be exiting Shriners. Finding all the coincidences with the number twenty-nine gave me reassurance and hope. It appeared there was some sort of plan in place, and I just needed to figure it out and follow it. Even if all the coincidences were just that – random coincidences – I took solace in them.

Living life with eczema had taught me patience, perseverance, and resilience. Overcoming it had been a marathon journey, but I had survived, thrived even. I knew I would also survive the job loss. I went to sleep that night, confident that my layoff would indeed have a silver lining.

COMFORT AND HOPE

Chapter 57

BY THE TIME Hurricane Irma hit Tampa on September 10, 2017, it had been downgraded to a Category 1. I stayed inside most of that day, watching the rain pelt the windows and high winds twist the trees outside my home. I had flashlights ready for the expected loss of power which surprisingly never came. The storm downed tree limbs, damaged some buildings, and caused flooding in some Tampa Bay areas, but I was lucky. My home was unscathed. As I sat curled on my couch after the storm had passed, I considered how, in just over a week's time, I had endured a layoff and a hurricane. I was eager to leave the turbulence of recent days behind and focus on my upcoming trip to Santa Fe.

On September 16, as I boarded the plane bound for New Mexico, I felt excited to explore a place I had never been to before. More importantly, getting away would give me time to relax and think about my future. The timing of the trip turned out to be perfect. I was looking forward to seeing my friend, who had also been laid off from Shriners a few years earlier. A great listener, she always had new ways of looking at things. I knew we would be comparing notes about our layoffs, and I wanted her input on how to move forward. We had both loved our jobs and faced challenges when our situations changed. She had reinvented herself professionally and it was my turn to do the same.

Arriving in Albuquerque, we got our rental car and headed out to Santa Fe. The drive was pleasant with very little traffic, and even though I was in unfamiliar territory I felt completely relaxed. Our beautiful Airbnb, decorated in typical southwest style with a hiking trail right behind it, was just perfect for us. The morning after we arrived, we hiked the scenic trail until it began to rain. We hurried back, showered, and headed into town. By then the rain had stopped and a gorgeous day stretched before us.

At our first stop downtown, we were able to find parking right near a famous Santa Fe landmark, the Catholic Cathedral Basilica of St. Francis of Assisi. The church, number one on our list of places to visit, was known for its stunning architecture. We grabbed our cameras and crossed the street to the front entrance.

There, directly in front of me, stood a life-sized statue of Saint Kateri Tekakwitha. I was surprised and amazed to see the statue thousands of miles from her birthplace and mine. I remembered the beautiful August day in 2009 when I had walked the grounds of the Kateri Shrine while in New York. I would never forget the peace I felt while soaking my hands in the cool spring water and praying for a cure for my eczema. It had been nearly eight years since I had any eczema on my hands. Of course, it was the primrose oil that had fixed the problem, but I would always wonder if Saint Kateri had also played a part in my relief.

The future felt so unsettled; seeing the statue brought comfort and hope. I thought about the many things I needed to do. Filing for unemployment, updating my resume, finding a new job, and buying health insurance were still huge tasks on my to-do list. And one other nagging item stubbornly remained on the list – finishing the book about my life with eczema. It had been a year and a half since *Spirituality and Health* magazine had published my letter and announced my forthcoming book. Yet I was not working on it at all. I still felt such a strong calling to tell my story, despite the fact that writing a book remained way out of my comfort zone.

Standing in front of Saint Kateri, I began to trust that things would work out for the best. Without a job, I would have plenty of time to complete the book and publish it.

And my voice would matter again.

SILVER LINING

Chapter 58

I ENJOYED THE rest of my trip to New Mexico, but a part of me was anxious to get back home to start the next chapter of my life – and the next chapter of my book. Back in Tampa, the thoughts pestering me to complete the book never stopped. After a few weeks, I logged onto the computer and forced myself to write, but I still lacked the discipline to get much done. I continued to work on the book in fits and starts for eight more months until I received some assistance from an unexpected source – my ballet class.

Often at the end of class, my fellow dance students and I would chat, not only about ballet, but also about our lives outside the studio. One day I discovered that another student, Elizabeth, had also experienced a recent layoff from a longtime job. It was comforting to connect with someone else who was in the same boat, struggling with the same issue at the same time.

"What kind of new job are you looking for?" I asked.

"Actually, I'm taking classes to earn my executive coach certification. And…I do need a lot of practice coaching hours to complete it, so if you know of anyone interested in being coached, just let me know," she replied.

In that moment, I had a hunch that meeting Elizabeth was a coincidence I could not ignore. I knew that coaching could help a person attain a personal or professional goal. She could obtain her coaching hours and I could finally finish writing my book. It was a ready-made win-win. I was sick of waking up at 4:00 in the morning, not with itching from eczema, but with the unfinished writing task weighing on my mind and disturbing my sleep. And yet in the light of day, I was frozen with insecurities and doubt about completing it. Having a coach would be a new experience for me and might be the extra help I needed to fully embrace the calling to share my story. With everything to gain, I decided to give it a try.

During our initial coaching session, Elizabeth asked me to consider what I might want to accomplish with coaching. I thought for half a second and then blurted out that I was writing a book and needed motivation to finish it. She seemed delighted with my ambition and I felt confident that she could help me. Not having to go it alone greatly reduced my stress level. Before I knew it, we had created a plan to jumpstart my temporarily stalled book and help me get back on track with my writing. Coaching provided support and encouragement and helped me persevere to reach my goal. Sometimes, in life, help came along exactly when it was needed.

A few weeks into coaching, I received another strong affirmation that I was on the right path in sharing my story. I had ordered more Efamol evening primrose oil, and when the bottles arrived I noticed that the packaging was different. The label was still bright yellow and blue, but instead of saying, "Pure Evening Primrose Oil Dietary Supplement," the product was labeled "Beautiful-Skin™ Evening Primrose Oil. Improve skin moisture, elasticity and firmness. Reduce roughness." But the best part was the last sentence: "Treat Eczema symptoms." I was pleased to see this stated right on the bottle.

I also realized that I never would have finished this book had I not been laid off. In a sense, my layoff was a blessing in disguise, freeing me to finally complete what I had started years before. If readers could relate to my book and perhaps be helped by it, then my goal would be achieved.

This finished book *is* my silver lining.

    ಚಿ   ಚಿ   ಚಿ

PART TWO

AFTER OVER FORTY years of experimenting with eczema treatments, I know a thing or two! In my quest to find answers, I researched eczema literature ad nauseum. In the sections following, you will find:

1. Thirty-six articles from a medical literature search on the use of evening primrose oil to treat eczema
2. My humble opinion of the medical research on evening primrose oil and eczema
3. Further online research from the National Eczema Association
4. Treatments and medications that I used for my eczema over a forty-five-year period
5. Claire's Top Ten List of Eczema Suggestions
6. "Itch, Scratch, *Relief*"
7. Notes

MEDICAL LITERATURE SEARCH ON THE USE OF EVENING PRIMROSE OIL TO TREAT ECZEMA: 36 ARTICLES

AS A MEDICAL librarian, I frequently performed literature searches on PubMed (https://www.ncbi.nlm.nih.gov/pubmed/), which is the free database from the National Library of Medicine. This database lists citations and abstracts on health and medicine and is used by physicians, researchers, and others in the medical field, as well as medical librarians. It is one of the best places to find the latest advances and research in medicine. A search for "(eczema OR atopic dermatitis) AND primrose oil" produced a list of articles discussing the use of evening primrose oil for treating eczema, and also brought up articles where the authors referred to eczema as "atopic dermatitis." There are many ways to design a literature search and the results can vary greatly, as literature searching is not an exact science.

In the thirty-six references listed below, you will see that the research is indeed controversial and fraught with at least some bit of disagreement. The first five articles in this list, published in the

1980s and early 1990s, were written by the same group of researchers: Drs. Horrobin, Lovell, Burton, Wright, Manku, and Morse. They all agreed that patients taking oral evening primrose oil all saw improvement in their eczema symptoms. Then it got interesting. Different researchers conducted other studies and found no improvement in eczema symptoms. A battle then ensued between advocates of primrose oil and those against it. It appears that this battle is still going on today, with some of the same players.

I have provided a brief description of each article, as well as some of my own thoughts on the research, which appear below each citation. You will need to draw your own conclusion, but perhaps you can gain some insight and alternate perspectives from the medical literature that follows.

1. TREATMENT OF ATOPIC ECZEMA WITH EVENING PRIMROSE OIL.

Lovell CR, Burton JL, Horrobin DF.
Lancet 1981 Jan 31; 1(8214):278.
PMID: 6109930

This 1981 article was one of the first published in the medical literature that discussed the value of oral evening primrose oil in the treatment of eczema. One of the authors was David Horrobin, MD, who was a major proponent of using evening primrose oil to treat several medical conditions. He was born in England and studied at Oxford, receiving degrees in medicine, neurophysiology, and neuroendocrinology. He founded Efamol, a company that produces evening primrose oil.

As a librarian, I felt a connection to Dr. Horrobin, as he first experimented with the use of evening primrose oil for eczema with the son of a librarian at his college. His work helped both the librarian's son and me!

2. ORAL EVENING-PRIMROSE-SEED OIL IMPROVES ATOPIC ECZEMA.

Wright S, Burton JL.
Lancet. 1982 Nov 20; 2(8308):1120-2.
PMID: 6128449

This was the original study that first prompted me to try the primrose oil to treat my eczema. The Redbook magazine article that I found in July 1983 referred to this study, which was published in November 1982 in the journal Lancet.

3. REDUCED LEVELS OF PROSTAGLANDIN IN PRECURSORS IN THE BLOOD OF ATOPIC PATIENTS: DEFECTIVE DELTA-6-DE-SATURASE FUNCTION AS A BIOCHEMICAL BASIS FOR ATOPY.

Manku MS, Horrobin DF, Morse N, Kyte
V, Jenkins K, Wright S, Burton JL.
Prostaglandins, Leukotrienes, and medicine. 1982 Dec; 9(6):615-28.
PMID: 6961468

This study looked at fifty patients (young adults) with eczema. The authors suggested that persons with eczema have a defect in the functioning of an enzyme (delta-6-desaturase) that converts the cis-linoleic acid to gamma-linolenic acid. They noted that all the patients had an elevation of cis-linoleic acid along with a deficit of gamma-linolenic acid. This defect in the enzyme functioning may have been the cause of the eczema. Evening primrose oil may act as this enzyme and help to correct this defect, thereby lessening or eliminating the eczema. Drs. Horrobin, Wright, and Burton are among the authors once again.

4. ESSENTIAL FATTY ACIDS IN THE PLASMA PHOS-PHOLIPIDS OF PATIENTS WITH ATOPIC ECZEMA.

Manku MS, Horrobin DF, Morse NL, Wright S, Burton JL.
British Journal of Dermatology. 1984 Jun; 110(6):643-8.
PMID: 6329254

This study, also by Horrobin, Wright, and Burton, viewed eczema as a defect in an enzyme (delta-6-desaturase), which resulted in abnormal metabolism. Oral supplementation with evening primrose oil helped to correct this metabolic abnormality.

5. ATOPIC DERMATITIS AND ESSENTIAL FATTY ACIDS: A BIOCHEMICAL BASIS FOR ATOPY?

Wright S.
Acta Dermato-venereologica. Supplementum. 1985; 114:143-5.
PMID: 3890448

A Swedish study of ninety-nine patients echoed the earlier studies that eczema is caused by an abnormality in the enzyme delta-6-desaturase. It reinforced the finding that evening primrose oil could improve eczema.

6. ATOPIC ECZEMA UNRESPONSIVE TO EVENING PRIMROSE OIL (LINOLEIC AND GAMMA-LINOLENIC ACIDS).

Bamford JT, Gibson RW, Renier CM.
Journal of the American Academy of Dermatology. 1985 Dec; 13(6):959-65.
PMID: 3908514

The research started to get more intriguing with the publication of this article! This was one of the first studies to disagree with prior studies that primrose oil is helpful to eczema sufferers. The authors looked at 123 patients with eczema and gave them varying doses of primrose oil. According to this group of researchers, the primrose oil did not help.

7. EVENING PRIMROSE OIL IN THE TREATMENT OF ATOPIC ECZEMA: EFFECT ON CLINICAL STATUS, PLASMA PHOSPHOLIPID FATTY ACIDS AND CIRCULATING BLOOD PROSTAGLANDINS.

Schalin-Karrila M, Mattila L, Jansen CT, Uotila P.

British Journal of Dermatology. 1987 Jul; 117(1):11-9.
Source: Department of Physiology, University of Turku, Finland.
PMID: 3307886

This study from Finland, by a different group of researchers, saw improvement in eczema symptoms. Participants took primrose oil for twelve weeks, and as a result had much less dryness and itching.

8. A LONG-TERM STUDY ON THE USE OF EVENING PRIMROSE OIL (EFAMOL) IN ATOPIC CHILDREN.

Biagi PL, Bordoni A, Masi M, Ricci G, Fanelli C, Patrizi A, Ceccolini E. *Drugs Under Experimental and Clinical Research.* 1988; 14(4):285-90.
Source: Nutrition Research Centre, University of Bologna, Italy.
PMID: 3048952

In a study from Italy, by yet another group of researchers, it was noted that a controversy was brewing over the effectiveness of the primrose oil on eczema. They conducted their own study on a group of children with eczema. After four weeks of taking primrose oil, the children's symptoms were dramatically improved. The group took primrose oil for another sixteen weeks and continued to show improvement.

9. EVENING PRIMROSE OIL (EFAMOL) IN THE TREATMENT OF CHILDREN WITH ATOPIC ECZEMA.

Bordoni A, Biagi PL, Masi M, Ricci G, Fanelli C, Patrizi A, Ceccolini E. *Drugs Under Experimental and Clinical Research.* 1988; 14(4):291-7.
Source: Nutrition Research Centre, University of Bologna, Italy.
PMID: 3048953

This article, by the same authors as article #8 above, reiterated that primrose oil is effective in treating eczema in both adults and children.

10. META-ANALYSIS OF PLACEBO-CONTROLLED STUDIES OF THE EFFICACY OF EPOGAM IN THE TREATMENT OF ATOPIC ECZEMA. RELATIONSHIP BETWEEN PLASMA ESSENTIAL FATTY ACID CHANGES AND CLINICAL RESPONSE.

Morse PF, Horrobin DF, Manku MS, Stewart JC, Allen R, Littlewood S, Wright S, Burton J, Gould DJ, Holt PJ, et al.
British Journal of Dermatology. 1989 Jul; 121(1):75-90.
Source: Efamol Research Institute, Woodbridge
Meadows, Guildford, UK.
PMID: 2667620

Another article by primrose oil's advocates, Dr. Horrobin and his colleagues at the Efamol Research Institute, highlighted the successful use of primrose oil in treating eczema. Nine controlled trials were discussed, in which participants' eczema was improved by primrose oil. Most noticeable was the oil's effect on reducing the intense itching.

Reducing the itching was the most important outcome for me. Nothing relieved the itching except the primrose oil. It was interesting to note that two of my friends with eczema who did not have as much itching were not helped by the primrose oil.

11. THE EFFECTS OF EVENING PRIMROSE OIL, SAFFLOWER OIL AND PARAFFIN ON PLASMA FATTY ACID LEVELS IN HUMANS: CHOICE OF AN APPROPRIATE PLACEBO FOR CLINICAL STUDIES ON PRIMROSE OIL.

Horrobin DF, Ells KM, Morse-Fisher N, Manku MS.
Prostaglandins Leukotrienes and Essential Fatty Acids. 1991 Apr; 42(4):245-9.
Source: Efamol Research Institute, Kentville, Nova Scotia, Canada.
PMID: 1871175

This 1991 study, conducted by Efamol and Dr. Horrobin, focused on finding an appropriate placebo to use when studying the effects of primrose oil. It appeared that even the studies on finding an effective placebo reached different conclusions and became controversial.

12. SUPPLEMENTATION WITH EVENING PRIMROSE OIL IN ATOPIC DERMATITIS: EFFECT ON FATTY ACIDS IN NEUTROPHILS AND EPIDERMIS.

Schäfer L, Kragballe K.
Lipids. 1991 Jul; 26(7):557-60.
Source: Aarhus Oliefabrik A/S, Research Laboratories, Denmark.
PMID: 1943500

Research from Denmark divided patients into three groups, giving each group a different dose of evening primrose oil to treat eczema. The authors theorized that abnormal lipid and fatty acid levels contributed to eczema, and that supplementation with evening primrose oil was a good way to balance out these levels. They determined that a higher dose of primrose oil was the most beneficial.

13. TREATMENT OF ATOPIC ECZEMA WITH EVENING PRIMROSE OIL: RATIONALE AND CLINICAL RESULTS.

Kerscher MJ, Korting HC.
The Clinical Investigator. 1992 Feb; 70(2):167-71.
Source: Dermatologische Klinik und Poliklinik
Ludwig-Maximilians Universität München.
PMID: 1318129

This article from Germany echoed earlier studies that some people may have a defect in the functioning of a particular enzyme (delta-6-desaturase), and this defect may cause them to develop eczema at some point. The primrose oil acted as this enzyme to lessen the symptoms of eczema. Participants who took the primrose oil had less itching, dryness, and scaling. The authors also added that primrose oil appeared safe, but more studies were needed.

14. PLACEBO-CONTROLLED TRIAL OF ESSENTIAL FATTY ACID SUPPLEMENTATION IN ATOPIC DERMATITIS.

Berth-Jones J, Graham-Brown RA.
Lancet. 1993 Jun; 19:341(8860):1557-60.
Source: Department of Dermatology,
Leicester Royal Infirmary, UK.

Authors of this study, Berth-Jones and Graham-Brown of the UK, conducted a study using a different methodology from prior studies, and concluded that primrose oil does not work for eczema.

15. THE EFFECT OF GAMMA-LINOLENIC ACID ON CLINICAL STATUS, RED CELL FATTY ACID COMPOSITION AND MEMBRANE MICROVISCOSITY IN INFANTS WITH ATOPIC DERMATITIS.

Biagi PL, Bordoni A, Hrelia S, Celadon M, Ricci GP, Cannella V, Patrizi A, Specchia F, Masi M.
Drugs Under Experimental and Clinical Research. 1994; 20(2):77-84.
Source: Department of Biochemistry G. Moruzzi, University of Bologna, Italy.
PMID: 7924900

This study from Italy tested primrose oil on a group of preschool children with eczema. Researchers also tested the children for allergies. They found that the primrose oil reduced the eczema in all the children, whether or not the children had allergies.

16. EPOGAM EVENING PRIMROSE OIL TREATMENT IN ATOPIC DERMATITIS AND ASTHMA.

Hederos CA, Berg A.
Archives of Disease in Childhood. 1996 Dec; 75(6):494-7.
Source: Paediatric Clinic, Health Centre, Gripen, Karlstad, Sweden.
PMID: 9014601

Swedish researchers investigated the use of primrose oil with sixty children who had eczema. Of the sixty children, twenty-two also had asthma. Participants took either Epogam evening primrose oil capsules or a placebo for sixteen weeks. The study showed great improvement of eczema symptoms in the group taking the primrose capsules, but no improvement in the placebo group. The children who also had asthma saw no improvement in their asthma symptoms.

Although I did not have asthma, over the years many of my dermatologists asked me about it, as this condition sometimes exists together with eczema. It was interesting to see a primrose oil study that addressed both of these issues at the same time.

17. PHARMACOKINETIC DATA OF GAMMA-LINOLE-NIC ACID IN HEALTHY VOLUNTEERS AFTER THE ADMINISTRATION OF EVENING PRIMROSE OIL (EPOGAM).

Martens-Lobenhoffer J, Meyer FP.
International Journal of Clinical Pharmacology and Therapeutics. 1998 Jul; 36(7):363-6.
Source: Institute of Clinical Pharmacology, University Hospital, Magdeburg, Germany.
PMID: 9707349

This study from Germany measured various levels of fatty acids, before and after administration of evening primrose oil to persons who did not have eczema. The research concluded that more studies were needed to determine whether or not primrose oil would help patients with eczema.

18. EFFECT OF TOPICALLY APPLIED EVENING PRIMROSE OIL ON EPIDERMAL BARRIER FUNCTION IN ATOPIC DERMATITIS AS A FUNCTION OF VEHICLE.

Gehring W, Bopp R, Rippke F, Gloor M.
Arzneimittel-Forschung. 1999 Jul; 49(7):635-42.

Source: Dermatology Clinic, Klinikum der Stadt
Karlsruhe gGmbH, Karlsruhe, Germany.
PMID: 10442214

Participants were asked to apply evening primrose oil onto their
skin (topically) in this study from Germany. Researchers concluded that it was helpful if a certain type of emulsion was used
with the primrose oil.

I never tried applying evening primrose oil to my skin. I was tired
of applying creams and lotions to my hands. I chose to eliminate my
eczema from the inside. But perhaps applying the oil topically provided some relief for folks who had an aversion to taking capsules.

19. SYSTEMATIC REVIEW OF TREATMENTS FOR ATOPIC ECZEMA.

Hoare C, Li Wan Po A, Williams H.
Health Technology Assessment 2000; 4(37):1-191.
Source: Centre of Evidence-Based Dermatology, University of
Nottingham, Queens Medical Centre NHS Trust, Nottingham, UK.
PMID: 11134919

This paper, published in 2000, examined 1165 randomized controlled studies on eczema treatments. The UK authors eliminated
893 of these studies due to a lack of appropriate data. They examined the remaining 272 studies, which contained 47 possible treatments for eczema. The researchers concluded that steroid creams,
ultraviolet light, and psychotherapy worked. Other treatments
such as Chinese herbs and primrose oil did not.

20. THE THERAPEUTIC EFFECT OF EVENING PRIM-ROSE OIL IN ATOPIC DERMATITIS PATIENTS WITH DRY SCALY SKIN LESIONS IS ASSOCIATED WITH THE NORMAL-IZATION OF SERUM GAMMA-INTERFERON LEVELS.

Yoon S, Lee J, Lee S.

Skin Pharmacology and Applied Skin Physiology 2002 Jan-Feb; 15(1):20-5.
Source: Department of Dermatology, College of Medicine, Inha University, Inchon, Republic of Korea.
PMID: 11803254

A Korean study tested primrose oil on fourteen patients with a certain type of eczema, the itchy, dry, scaly type. After treatment, itching was reduced significantly in all patients. They concluded that evening primrose oil was very helpful in the treatment of a "non-inflammatory" type of atopic dermatitis.

21. TREATMENT OF CHILDHOOD ECZEMA.

Granlund H.
Paediatric Drugs 2002; 4(11):729-35.
Source: Department of Dermatology, Helsinki University Central Hospital, Helsinki, Finland.
PMID: 12390044

This article from Finland discussed the most common treatments for eczema, such as emollients and steroid creams. The author listed many alternative treatments including evening primrose oil, Chinese herbs, and oral antihistamines, but stated that these treatments had not been studied properly; therefore, there was no firm evidence of their effectiveness.

22. THE USE OF DIETARY MANIPULATION BY PARENTS OF CHILDREN WITH ATOPIC DERMATITIS.

Johnston GA, Bilbao RM, Graham-Brown RA.
British Journal of Dermatology. 2004 Jun; 150(6):1186-9.
Source: Department of Dermatology, Leicester Royal Infirmary, LE1 5WW, UK.
PMID: 15214908

A United Kingdom study included interviews with 100 parents who had tried various diets to control their child's eczema. A few parents eliminated dairy products, including milk, and eggs. Fifty-nine percent of parents supplemented their child's diet with evening primrose oil and of these, 13% felt their child's skin improved.

Only half of the parents consulted a physician before trying any of these diet changes or supplementation.

23. A REVIEW OF THE CLINICAL EFFICACY OF EVENING PRIMROSE.

Stonemetz D.
Holistic Nursing Practice 2008 May-Jun; 22(3):171-4.
Source: OB/GYN Associates of Western New York, West Seneca, NY 14224, USA. ds465@drexel.edu
PMID: 18453897

A review article from the US mentioned that evening primrose oil is rich in omega-6 fatty acids, which are necessary for many processes in the body. The article noted that the oil was used for eczema and also mastalgia (breast tenderness or pain). It was concluded that there was a lack of evidence to support either of these treatment options.

24. WHAT'S NEW IN ATOPIC ECZEMA? AN ANALYSIS OF THE CLINICAL SIGNIFICANCE OF SYSTEMATIC REVIEWS ON ATOPIC ECZEMA PUBLISHED IN 2006 AND 2007.

Williams HC, Grindlay DJ.
Clinical and Experimental Dermatology. 2008 Nov; 33(6):685-8.
Source: National Library for Health Skin Disorders Specialist Library, Centre of Evidence-Based Dermatology, University of Nottingham.
PMID: 18691244

This review paper summarized studies on eczema that were published in 2006 and 2007. The authors discovered that families with children who have eczema could benefit from educational support. They stated that there was little evidence that evening primrose oil was helpful, but more studies were needed.

25. EVENING PRIMROSE OIL IS EFFECTIVE IN ATOPIC DERMATITIS: A RANDOMIZED PLACEBO-CONTROLLED TRIAL.

Senapati S, Banerjee S, Gangopadhyay DN.
Indian Journal of Dermatology, Venereology and Leprology. 2008 Sep-Oct; 74(5):447-52.
Source: Department of Dermatology, Calcutta National Medical College, Kolkata, India.
PMID: 19052401

Conducted in India, a study concluded that primrose oil was very effective in treating eczema and safe to take with no major side effects. Participants took primrose oil for five months. At the end of the fifth month, 96 percent of them showed marked improvement, and 32 percent of those taking a placebo showed some improvement. The authors felt that more studies needed to be done, since other researchers produced different results.

26. EVENING PRIMROSE OIL.

Bayles B, Usatine R.
American Family Physician. 2009 Dec 15; 80(12):1405-8.
Source: Dept. of Family and Community Medicine, University of Texas Health Science Center at San Antonio, 7703 Floyd Curl Dr., San Antonio, TX 78229.
PMID: 20000302

The authors proposed that most trials conducted using evening primrose oil to treat eczema had flaws in their methodology. They noted that primrose oil had few side effects, but warned that it should not be used during pregnancy. The authors discussed the use of the primrose oil for other health problems such as rheumatoid arthritis, premenstrual syndrome, and mastalgia (breast tenderness). They concluded that further studies were needed to determine effectiveness and proper dosing.

27. DIETARY SUPPLEMENTS FOR ESTABLISHED ATOPIC ECZEMA.

Bath-Hextall FJ, Jenkinson C, Humphreys R, Williams HC.
Cochrane Database of Systematic Reviews. 2012 Feb 15; 2.
Source: School of Nursing, Faculty of Medicine and Health Science, the University of Nottingham, Nottingham, UK.
PMID: 22336810

A 2012 study from England reviewed the literature on various dietary supplements as a treatment for eczema. It concluded that the evidence was sparse and supplements should not be recommended. The article looked at eleven studies with participants trying an array of supplements such as fish oil, vitamin D, vitamin E, and sunflower oil. These authors were not convinced of any benefit. They did not include primrose oil or borage oil in this study, as these oils were included in other Cochrane Reviews. This group of authors was open to more studies.

28. ORAL EVENING PRIMROSE OIL AND BORAGE OIL FOR ECZEMA.

Bamford JT, Ray S, Musekiwa A, van Gool C, Humphreys R, Ernst E.
Cochrane Database of Systematic Reviews. 2013 Apr 30; 4.
Source: Department of Family Medicine and Community Health, University of Minnesota Medical School, Duluth, Minnesota, USA.
PMID: 23633319

This study, appearing in the Cochrane Database of Systematic Reviews, searched the medical literature on evening primrose oil and borage oil in the treatment of eczema. The authors found nineteen studies on primrose oil and eight on borage oil and did an in-depth statistical analysis of these studies.

They searched databases and online trials registers, corresponding with pharmaceutical companies regarding other unpublished studies. The authors also searched side effects, and found one study that stated evening primrose oil might increase bleeding for people taking Coumadin. They stated that this review paper did not look at effects of long-term use, but mentioned a case report that suggested long-term use of evening primrose oil might cause inflammation, thrombosis, and immunosuppression. The authors concluded that alternative treatments such as evening primrose oil do not work and a case for future research would be difficult to defend.

This review paper made the news! It was highlighted in an email sent to physicians who subscribe to Medscape, which is produced by WebMD. A reference to this article and the resulting negative publicity about evening primrose oil also made the rounds on the internet. The New York Times mentioned the article in one of its columns, as did several other publications. The National Center for Complementary and Alternative Medicine also referred to it. Fortunately, consumers whose eczema had been helped by evening primrose oil responded to these negative claims with their own success stories. The comments section of various websites confirmed that evening primrose oil was helping at least a portion of folks who suffer from eczema.

I found this entire study to be quite ironic. The one and only treatment that ever actually worked for me was the very one these researchers emphatically stated did not work at all. Three points are particularly concerning to me:

1. POSSIBLE SIDE EFFECTS

The study mentioned that the use of primrose oil may possibly have side effects. Yet the steroid creams and other treatments that I tried caused multiple side effects. As an example, my long-term use of steroid creams caused thinning of the skin on my hands and striations (lines). The skin on the palms of my hands was so thin that my hands would get tiny cuts from picking up something that would not normally cause a cut in a person with normal skin. When I ceased using the steroid creams, my skin became stronger and thicker. I experienced absolutely no side effects from the primrose oil.

2. PHARMACEUTICAL COMPANIES' INFLUENCE

I found it unsettling that the authors included "unpublished" and "ongoing" studies from pharmaceutical companies to determine that primrose oil does not work. Pharmaceutical companies produce prescription drugs for eczema. If folks bought an over-the-counter, natural, herbal remedy for eczema that worked, they certainly would not need costly, prescription-only treatments. If physicians promoted evening primrose oil as an option, the pharmaceutical industry might lose a very profitable group of patients.

3. IMPLICATION THAT FURTHER RESEARCH ON PRIMROSE OIL WOULD BE DIFFICULT TO DEFEND

The Cochrane Database of Systematic Reviews reaches a wide audience, is highly credible, well respected, and trusted by the medical profession. But I was quite disheartened by the authors' implication that further research on primrose oil would be difficult to defend. Many other studies firmly state that evening primrose oil is helpful to some eczema patients. My runner friend and I are living proof of that.

If anything, MORE research is needed to determine which types of eczema may benefit from primrose oil, the most effective dosages, and long- or short-term side effects, if any.

I fully realize that evening primrose oil may not help every eczema patient. But shouldn't all those who deal with this maddening condition at least be given the knowledge that primrose oil could possibly help, so that they might try it and see for themselves?

29. EVENING PRIMROSE OIL AND BORAGE OIL DO NOT HELP ECZEMA SYMPTOMS, FINDS COCHRANE REVIEW.

Kmietowicz Z.
BMJ. 2013 Apr 29; 346:f2712.
PMID: 23628953

This article published in the prestigious BMJ journal is a recap of the Cochrane Database Systematic Review above (#28) restating firmly that evening primrose oil does not help eczema.

30. DOSE-DEPENDENT EFFECTS OF EVENING PRIMROSE OIL IN CHILDREN AND ADOLESCENTS WITH ATOPIC DERMATITIS.

Chung BY, Kim JH, Cho SI, Ahn IS, Kim HO, Park CW, Lee CH.
Annals of Dermatology 2013 Aug; 25(3):285-91.
Source: Department of Dermatology, Kangnam Sacred Heart Hospital, College of Medicine, Hallym University, Seoul, Korea.
PMID: 24003269

Authors of a Korean study aimed to determine the proper dosage of evening primrose oil that is needed to effectively treat eczema. It divided participants with eczema into two groups. One group was given a larger dose of evening primrose oil (320 mg twice daily for eight weeks) and the second group was given a smaller dose (160 mg daily for eight weeks). Both groups showed improvement in their eczema, but the group taking the larger dose showed greater improvement. Neither group had any side effects from the primrose oil.

More importantly, the participants in the study were not allowed to use any other treatments during the trial period, including steroid creams or picrolemus or tacrolemis. In fact, they had to stop all other treatments for several days to a few weeks before beginning to take the primrose oil.

This study supports my thoughts on the use of primrose oil on two counts. First, I had to take a higher dose consistently for several weeks (ten weeks to be exact) to see results. Secondly, I stopped the use of creams, lotions, and ointments for a few weeks before starting the primrose oil. All steroid creams, picrolemus, tacrolemis, and all over-the-counter ointments and creams had been completely stopped. It was only then that I was able to eliminate my eczema with the sole use of the evening primrose oil capsules.

31. GAMMA-LINOLENIC ACID LEVELS CORRELATE WITH CLINICAL EFFICACY OF EVENING PRIMROSE OIL IN PATIENTS WITH ATOPIC DERMATITIS.

Simon D, Eng PA, Borelli S, Kägi R, Zimmermann C, Zahner C, Drewe J, Hess L, Ferrari G, Lautenschlager S, Wüthrich B, Schmid-Grendelmeier P.
Advances in Therapy. 2014 Feb; 31(2):180-8.
PMID: 24435467

The study was done to determine which patients might benefit from evening primrose oil based on their level of gamma-linolenic acid, before and after primrose oil supplementation.

32. REVIEW OF EVIDENCE FOR DIETARY INFLU-ENCES ON ATOPIC DERMATITIS.

Mohajeri S, Newman SA.
Skin Therapy Letter. 2014 Jul-Aug; 19(4):5-7.
PMID: 25188523

The authors state that evening primrose oil supplementation, along with an omega-3 fatty acid, may help some people with atopic dermatitis.

33. WHAT'S NEW IN ATOPIC ECZEMA? AN ANALYSIS OF SYSTEMATIC REVIEWS PUBLISHED IN 2012 AND 2013. PART 2. TREATMENT AND PREVENTION.

Madhok V, Futamura M, Thomas KS, Barbarot S.
Clinical and Experimental Dermatology. 2015 Jun; 40(4):349-54.
PMID: 25622761

Based on two years (2012 and 2013) of published systematic reviews, the authors concluded that evening primrose oil and borage oil do not alleviate eczema.

34. DIET AND ECZEMA: A REVIEW OF DIETARY SUPPLEMENTS FOR THE TREATMENT OF ATOPIC DERMATITIS.

Schlichte MJ, Vandersall A, Katta R.
Dermatopathology Practical and Conceptual. 2016 Jul 31; 6(3)23-9.
PMID: 27648380

In this review paper, the authors stated that evening primrose oil and borage oil are no better than a placebo in treating eczema.

35. COMPLEMENTARY AND ALTERNATIVE MEDICINE FOR ATOPIC DERMATITIS: AN EVIDENCE-BASED REVIEW.

Vieira BL, Lim NR, Lohman Me, Lio PA.
American Journal of Clinical Dermatology. 2016 Dec; 17(6):557-581.
PMID: 27388911

This review article concluded that alternative medicine may work for atopic dermatitis, but more studies are needed. The authors mentioned evening primrose oil, hypnosis, stress reduction techniques, biofeedback, and vitamin D supplementation as well as some other alternative therapies that might offer relief.

Alternative medicine and herbal therapy are not going away. If anything, they are increasing in popularity. I hope that one day western medicine will fully embrace their possibilities.

36. EFFECT OF EVENING PRIMROSE OIL ON KOREAN PATIENTS WITH MILD ATOPIC DERMATITIS: A RANDOMIZED, DOUBLE-BLINDED, PLACEBO-CONTROLLED CLINICAL STUDY.

Chung BY, Park SY, Jung MJ, Kim HO, Park CW.
Annals of Dermatology. 2018 Aug; 30(4):409-416.
PMID: 30065580

This 2018 Korean study gave evening primrose oil capsules or a placebo to patients with mild eczema. Those taking the primrose oil showed marked improvement versus those taking a placebo. The authors reiterated the theory that atopic dermatitis is caused by a defect in the enzyme, delta-6-desaturase, and that evening primrose oil supplementation is helpful to correct this abnormality.

༂ ༂ ༂

MY HUMBLE OPINION OF THE MEDICAL RESEARCH RELATED TO EVENING PRIMROSE OIL AND ECZEMA

As you can see from my search of the medical literature, the study of evening primrose oil and eczema is very controversial and rampant with uncertainty. There are two distinct camps of researchers: those in favor and those against. Four decades after the first articles were published, there is still no strong conclusion. At last check, there were over forty thousand citations in the PubMed database on eczema/atopic dermatitis. Fewer than one hundred addressed the use of primrose oil to treat eczema. I firmly believe that more research is needed.

Some studies suggest that primrose oil works on the folks who have eczema caused by a defect in the enzyme delta-6-desaturase. If the eczema is caused by something else, then perhaps the primrose oil does not help. I had eczema mostly on my hands, which may have affected the success of this treatment in some way.

Hopefully, physicians will come to realize that what may not work for all, may indeed work for some, and is therefore at the very least worth mentioning. Patients need encouragement to try alternative treatments as well as traditional, standard treatments. The dermatologists that I visited over the years never once recommended primrose oil as a possible treatment. When I suggested it, they were skeptical. And looking at the medical literature, I can see why!

Primrose oil appears to be safe, with few or no side effects. If it works, that's great. If it doesn't, at least another possibility has been explored and can be ruled out. I am optimistic that for most patients there is some relief out there, be it a natural remedy or one of the more traditional treatments. I want to emphatically state that I am not against pharmaceuticals to treat eczema. If I still had it, I would be first in line to try the various new treatments, creams, and injections that are widely advertised, or even try to enroll in a clinical trial for a new study on eczema treatment. I am, however, very thankful that my eczema was eliminated by a plant-based herbal remedy which, for me, had no side effects.

FURTHER ONLINE RESEARCH: NATIONAL ECZEMA ASSOCIATION

In a Google search for eczema information, the National Eczema Association website (https://nationaleczema.org) appeared on the first page of results. The organization's home page stated that they "are the resource and the hub for the millions of Americans who are living with eczema."

As a medical librarian, I learned to evaluate websites objectively. At first glance, I found this website immediately useful, offering a great variety of resources for those diagnosed with eczema. One highlight of these resources was a list of over 240 eczema products such as creams, lotions, sunscreens, and even laundry detergents. It was valuable to have access to this long list of products all in one place. Many of them soothe the skin and provide some relief. However, if eczema were to become chronic these products may offer only temporary solutions. Other beneficial resources included facts about eczema, extensive research, a list of clinical trials, and an online support group. But a closer look at the site revealed that many pharmaceutical corporations were donating large sums of money to this association. This gave me pause, as these companies produced the drugs used to treat eczema.

As a result of these generous donations, was the entire website biased in their favor?

Alternative treatments, including evening primrose oil, lacked a favorable presence. The fear of possible unknown side effects from various alternative treatments emerged as a common theme on the website. But, ironically, many pharmaceutical preparations are proven to have unpleasant and potentially dangerous side effects. The effectiveness of alternative treatments was also questioned on the site. But it should be strongly noted that many widely advertised pharmaceutical products for eczema actually help only a small percentage of people, and carry known, unwanted side effects. At least the authors of the articles found on the website echoed my thoughts that much more research is needed on both the efficacy and possible side effects of alternative and non-traditional choices.

So how might these alternative treatments be evaluated more thoroughly and consistently by the contributors to the website?

As I previously stated, after forty years of eczema, I still support whatever might work to alleviate this condition for an individual. But it is not helpful to any of us seeking solutions when the focus of studies and research seems to gravitate toward pharmaceutical treatments instead of creating a balance of both traditional and alternative therapies. Neither offers a guarantee, but we need to study all the possibilities.

We could easily give in to the loudest voice, but at what cost?

TREATMENTS AND MEDICATIONS I USED FOR MY ECZEMA OVER A FORTY-FIVE-YEAR PERIOD

(Alphabetical List)

Acupuncture
Allegra 180
Allegra D12
Atarax
Atopiclair Nonsteroidal Cream
Aveeno Soothing Bath Treatment

Benadryl
Borage Oil
Brovex

Cetaphil Gentle Skin Cleanser
Cetaphil Moisturizing Cream
Clarinex-D 24 Hour (Desloratadine) 5mg
Clobex Topical Lotion (Clobetasol Propionate)

Cordran Tape (flurandrenolide)
Curel

Dead Sea Salt Psoriasis Cream
Decongestine Capsules (Chlorpheniramine/Pseudoephedrin)
Derma-Smoothe/FS Scalp Oil (Fluocinolone Acetonide 0.01% Topical Oil)
Dermatology Lotion
Dermatop Emollient Cream (Prednicarbate)
DesOwen
DHS Tar Shampoo
DHS Zinc Shampoo
Diprolene
Domeboro Astringent Solution (Aluminum Acetate)
Doxepin HCL 10mg

Elidel
Evening Primrose Oil

Florasone Cream (Cardiospermum Natural Homeopathic)
Fluocinolone Acetonide Ointment USP 0.025%

Hot Water
Hydrocortisone Cream 2.5%
Hydroxyzine HCL Tab 25 mg
Hypnosis
Hytone

Kenalog Cream

Lidex-E (Fluocinonide)
Light Box

Malena
Medical Radiation (Roentgen therapy)
Mimyx Cream

Oil of oregano
Oilatum Cleansing Bar
Olux Foam 0.05% (Clobetasol Propionate)

Palgic
Prednisone
Protopic

Rynatan (Phenylephrine Tannate 25 mg,
Chlorpheniramine Tannate, 9 mg)

Sarna Original Anti-Itch Lotion
Scalpicin
Seldane
Seldane D
Singulair 10 mg Tablets (Montelukast Sodium)
Sudafed 12 Hour

Vaseline Petroleum Jelly
Vanos (Fluocinonide Cream 0.1%)

Westcort

Zoloft
Zyrtec Tab 10mg

CLAIRE'S TOP TEN LIST OF ECZEMA SUGGESTIONS

1. Know that you are not alone. Eczema is very common.
2. Keep an open mind to explore options. What works for one person may not work for another.
3. Make sure the dermatologist you visit specializes in eczema (a lesson learned the hard way – see Chapter 35).
4. Try the treatment for the length of time recommended, unless you seem to be allergic to it or it is making the eczema worse (also learned the hard way – see Chapter 44).
5. Follow the directions exactly unless your doctor suggests otherwise.
6. Buy high quality products even if they are more expensive. Why take the chance that the cheaper version will work as well? Once your eczema is under control you can experiment with other brands.
7. Try ONE treatment at a time. If you try too many at once, you will not know which one is working. Also, some treatments done together may cancel each other out.
8. Keep a log of treatments, dates used, and results. This will help both you and your health care provider track your progress.

9. Continue to educate yourself on current eczema treatments. Read, study, research, and join communities of interest, either online or in person.

10. Think of eczema as a challenge. You can rise above it. Don't give up!

ITCH. SCRATCH. *RELIEF.*

My eczema life could fill up a book
Itching and scratching wherever I look.
The creams, they were useless and made me insane
Wrinkling my skin, too many to name.

I tried all the treatments till blue in the face
My hands were still bloody, no help in this case.
I went to the doctor each month of the year.
None were of help, which was always my fear.

But they tried, and they tried yet again and again.
Steroids, more steroids, will this ever end?
Lastly, I'd had it and was ready to quit.
When finally, one day I found the right fit.

The oil that I used was not fancy or fine.
Just mellow and smooth, much like a good wine.
Easy to swallow and cheap on the dime,
It cured what had ailed me, all in good time.

So now days are brighter, the sun always shines.
My life without scratching is frankly divine.
The itching is gone, with its fury and wrath
Now that I saunter the calm primrose path.

NOTES

FOREWORD

The reference to the incidence of eczema comes from "Atopic dermatitis: Global epidemiology and risk factors," S Nutten, *Annals of Nutrition and Metabolism* 66 Suppl 1 (2015):8-16.

The statement on atopic dermatitis being a lifelong illness was quoted from "Persistence of mild to moderate atopic dermatitis," JS Margolis et al., *JAMA Dermatology* 150 (2014): 593-600.

PART ONE
CHAPTER 6

The use of medical radiation in treating eczema was taken from "The value of roentgen therapy in dermatology," GM MacKee et al., *American Journal of Roentgenology and Radium Therapy* 9 (1922): 241-246, and the article by MB Sulzberger et al., "Do Roentgen-Ray treatments as given by skin specialists produce cancers or other sequelae?" *American Medical Association Archives of Dermatology and Syphilology* 65 (1952): 639-655.

It is also discussed in detail in the book by GM MacKee, *XRays and Radium in the Treatment of Diseases of the Skin*. Malvern, PA: Lea & Febiger, 1938.

CHAPTER 7

The study on secondhand smoke and eczema came from "The effect of environmental tobacco smoke on eczema and allergic sensitization in children," U Kramer et al., *British Journal of Dermatology* 150 (2004): 111–118.

CHAPTER 9

The reference to cholesterol testing in children is taken from "Cholesterol testing among children and adolescents during health visits," SR Vinci et al., *JAMA 311 (*2014): 1804-7.

CHAPTER 14

Chlorine and eczema were taken from "Swimming pools and eczema," J Van Onselen, *Journal of Family Health* Suppl (2015) 8-9.

CHAPTER 17

The information on eczema and hot, humid climates is taken from "Warm, humid, and high sun exposure climates are associated with poorly controlled eczema: PEER (Pediatric Eczema Elective Registry) cohort, 2004-2012," by MR Sarten et al., *Journal of Investigative Dermatology* 134 (2014): 51-7.

CHAPTER 21

Stress causing increased itching of eczema is from "Impact of acute stress on itch sensation and scratching behaviour in patients with atopic dermatitis and healthy controls," H Mochizuki et al., *British Journal of Dermatology* 180 (2019): 821-827.

CHAPTER 22

Steroid side effects are mentioned in "Possible side effects of topical steroids," MR Morman, *American Family Physician* 23 (1981):171-4.

Dermatologists' recommendation to moisturize dry eczematous skin is from "Treatment with a barrier-strengthening moist cream delays relapse of atopic dermatitis: a prospective and randomized controlled clinical trial," by K Wiren et al., *Journal of the European Academy of Dermatology and Venereology* 23 (2009):1267-72.

CHAPTER 23

The Redbook article mentioned is from "Flower Power: evening primrose oil," by Dianne Hales, *Redbook* July (1983), 29.

CHAPTER 33

The use of acupuncture and Chinese herbal medicine in treating atopic dermatitis is mentioned in "The effectiveness of combined Chinese herbal medicine and acupuncture in the treatment of atopic dermatitis," by F Salameh et al., *Journal of Alternative and Complementary Medicine* 14 (2008):1043-8.

CHAPTER 41

The use of hypnosis to treat eczema and atopic dermatitis was taken from "Hypnotherapy as a treatment for atopic dermatitis in adults and children," by AC Stewart, *British Journal of Dermatology* 132 (1995):778-83.

CHAPTER 43

The statement about lemon-scented detergent and hot water irritating the skin of dishwashers in Denmark was taken from "Temperature dependent primary irritant dermatitis from lemon perfume," by HW Rothenberg, *Contact Dermatitis* 3 (1977):37-48.

CHAPTER 56

The description of the near-death experience is taken from Meo, Patricia, "A near-death experience," *Nursing Spectrum, Florida Edition*, 9 (1999):4.

The meaning of the number 29 is taken from Jones, Stephen E., *The Biblical Meaning of Numbers (Genesis Book of Psalms 2)*, God's Kingdom Ministries, 2008.

PART TWO
MEDICAL LITERATURE SEARCH ON THE USE OF EVENING PRIMROSE OIL TO TREAT ECZEMA: 36 ARTICLES

The statement on evening primrose oil not helping eczema was taken from "Eczema: Evening Primrose Oil, Borage Oil Not Helpful" *Medscape*, Apr 29, 2013.

The statement about negative publicity was taken from "Really? The Claim: Evening Primrose Oil Helps Eczema," by Anahad O'Connor, *New York Times*, April 29, 2013.

FURTHER ONLINE RESEARCH: NATIONAL ECZEMA ASSOCIATION

https://nationaleczema.org/
Accessed April 2020

Printed in Great Britain
by Amazon